The Rogue Librarian's Guide To Sleep— Real Help for Insomnia

By Will Swartz

The Rogue Librarian's Guide To Sleep

This book is a work of the author's expertise and experience. While every effort has been made to ensure the accuracy of the information presented, the author and publisher make no warranties or representations regarding its completeness or applicability. The information provided is for educational and informational purposes only and should not be considered medical, psychological, or legal advice. Readers should consult with a qualified professional for specific guidance related to their situation. The author and publisher assume no responsibility for errors, omissions, or the use or misuse of the information contained herein.

Any trademarks mentioned are the property of their respective owners and are used only for reference, without any affiliation or endorsement implied.

Printed in the USA.
First Edition

ISBN (Print): 978-0-9967932-3-0

For more information, visit

https://linktr.ee/wswartz

Bonus Sleep Toolkit

Hey Sleepless Reader...

Before you dive in headfirst and finally get the rest you deserve (and honestly, need), I've got a gift for you.

It's called **The Rogue Librarian's Sleep Toolkit**, and it's completely free. Think of it like the Swiss Army Knife of bedtime. You'll get:

- Downloadable checklists

- Worksheets to help you build your perfect sleep routine

- Tracking tools (not creepy ones, just the helpful kind)

- Links to gadgets, gear, and resources I personally recommend

And a few delightful surprises I couldn't squeeze into this book. All of it lives on one simple, beautiful,insomnia-busting page.

Why am I giving this away? Because two things are true:

1. I want you to sleep better. Really. That's the whole point.

2. I'd love to send you even more Rogue wisdom, stories, and practical tools to help with sleep and other things we humans tend to mess up.

No spam. Just me (and my over caffeinated brain) occasionally dropping something helpful, funny, or potentially life-improving into your inbox

So go ahead—scan the code. Get the goods.

And let's get you sleeping like a Hemingway cat.

To Noah, Noelle, Jeremy, Josiah, and Jennifer—

For every sleepless night you so generously provided, whether through midnight feedings, irrational toddler demands, or the sudden and urgent need to explain the mysteries of the universe at 2 AM. For the early morning practices that turned me into a sleep-deprived chauffeur. For the late-night games, last-minute school projects, and inexplicable bursts of energy when I was running on fumes.

You all made sure I had a front-row seat to the many ways a person can be deprived of sleep, and I'd like to think that hands-on experience gave me the credentials to write this book.

I wouldn't trade a single exhausted moment for the world (though I might have traded a few for a solid nap). You are, and always will be, my greatest adventure—even if you did rob me of a few thousand hours of rest along the way.

With love, yawns, and the eternal hope that you're all getting better sleep than I did,

—Dad

Table of Contents

A Rogue Librarian's Guide to Sleep 1

Sleep Triage—Start Here! 5

The Mysterious, Necessary Superpower 7

The Most Bizarre, Hilarious, and Fascinating
Sleep Remedies Ever Devised 16

Sleep Temples, Hammocks, and the Delusions of
Ancient Insomniacs 17

Melatonin: The Sandman's Little Helper or Just
Another Sleepy Time Myth? 27

Cutting Edge Pharmacological Sleep Solutions:
Beyond Counting Sheep 32

The Digital Insomniac's Dilemma.....................37

The Truth About Insomnia (And Why You Can
Fix It) 44

Earn Your Sleep: Move More 52

Bedroom Benefits: How Sex and Sleep Are
Secretly Best Friends...58

Eating Your Way to Better Sleep—or the
Midnight Snack That Ruined Everything.......63

Your Bedroom Called… 73

Breaking The "Tired But Wired" Cycle..........83

The "Mind Off" Formula – Stopping Racing Thoughts At Night 90

The Military Method: Falling Asleep Like a Soldier 100

The 5-Step Nighttime Routine That Signals "Sleep Mode" 107

How I Sleep Like Hemingway's Cats in the Sunshine 112

The End of the Book, but Not the End of Your Journey 125

Bonus Chapter: What to Do When You STILL Can't Sleep 128

About the author....................................137

Also by Will Swartz 140

A Rogue Librarian's Guide to Sleep

L et's get something straight right away: I'm not that kind of librarian.

You know the type—the tight bun, the icy glare over the rim of some bedazzled spectacles, the ever-raised finger ready to shush even the slightest sound. Nope, I'm more of a rogue librarian, the kind who believes books should be touched, information is meant to be shared, (not hoarded), and that research is an adventure, not a chore. And, lucky for you, my latest deep dive has been into something we all desperately want more of: sleep.

This book is the result of my obsessive curiosity about how to fall asleep faster and stay asleep longer. I wish I had written it years ago, when I first became a parent. It all started with a single question: Could I train myself to fall asleep in two minutes? I had heard about a method developed by the military —something designed to help soldiers sleep in any condition, even under battlefield stress. That was enough to send me tumbling down the rabbit hole, and I emerged weeks later with stacks of research, studies, personal trials, and a much deeper understanding of what works—and what doesn't—when it comes to sleep.

If there's one thing you should know about me, it's this: I don't do shallow research. I dive into the deep end and swim for the bottom. I verify. I cross-reference. And I don't just parrot dry studies—I translate them into something you can actually *use*. Because honestly, what good is knowledge if it doesn't help you solve a problem? That's why this book is for real people—not scientists in lab coats or sleep specialists who speak fluent jargon.

My goal? Make this practical, engaging, and—most importantly—effective. And maybe entertain you a bit, too.

Sleep is one of life's essentials—and yet, so many of us wrestle with it. I know this firsthand. I've been that guy, fighting to keep his eyes open in meetings —too tired to think straight but somehow still too wired to sleep at night. I've known the bone-deep exhaustion of trying to juggle work, exercise, nutrition, family time, relaxation, and a strong spiritual connection. All while raising five kids, running on fumes and caffeine, and wondering if I'd ever feel truly rested again.

I've also wandered through the frustrating maze of sleep apnea. The late-night tossing and turning. The constant fatigue no amount of coffee could fix. Sleep studies. The doctor visits. And the special moment when I was told, "You stop breathing 69 times per hour in your sleep." (Fun times.)

Adapting to a CPAP machine felt like trying to sleep in a scuba mask—with a jet engine strapped to your face. Let's just say, it wasn't exactly love at first breath. I know what it's like to wrestle with change, to try everything under the sun (and moon) just to get a decent night's sleep.

Whatever your battle with sleep looks like—racing mind at 2 AM, slow torture of sleep deprivation, or the sheer frustration of knowing something's wrong but having no clue how to fix it—this book is here to change that. Not with quick fixes or gimmicks, but with real, practical strategies that actually work. Because if I can find my way to better sleep, I promise you can too.

Through science-backed methods, real-world hacks, and a bit of humor along the way, I'll show you how to take back control of your sleep. Because as it turns out, better sleep isn't just a dream—it's something you can *learn, train for,* and *master.* By the time you finish this book, you'll know exactly what to do to fall asleep faster, stay asleep longer, and wake up feeling more rested — without gimmicks or guesswork.

Sleep Triage—Start Here!

Y ou're desperate for sleep. Trust me—I get it. You don't need a deep dive into the mystical world of sleep science, a dissertation on circadian rhythms, or a 27-page PDF proving that blue light is the bogeyman lurking in your phone. If I start waving around a stack of studies, you'll be gone faster than I can say "melatonin."

No, what you want—what you *need*—is someone to cut through the noise and just *tell you what to do*. **Right now!**

Fine. Here's the deal: Read these two chapters— *Earn Your Sleep* and *The Military Method*.

Then come back to read the rest of the book.

These two chapters are the best advice I can give you for quick wins and will give you something practical to do right now.

Yes, the rest of this book is full of useful stuff— things that might actually change your relationship with sleep forever. These two chapters? They're what I'd shout at you if we were stuck in an elevator and had 30 seconds before the doors opened.

So read them. And if you're too tired to read? Have someone read them to you. Or print them out and sleep on them. Whatever it takes. Just start with those two chapters and then come back here when you're rested.

For those still here, I've arranged this book in a logical order but you can use the table of contents to jump to individual chapters on different topics related to sleep.

There's a Sleep Research Resources section at the end of the book if you're the curious type who wants to dig deeper.

The Mysterious, Necessary Superpower

"Sleep is like a cat: it only comes to you if you ignore it." — Gillian Flynn

M ost people think of sleep as that annoying thing that cuts the day in half. You get tired, you flop over, you're unconscious for a while, you get up, you go. Rinse and repeat. But under the hood, sleep is one of the most complex, vital, and frankly astonishing things your body and mind do all day—and night.

Sleep isn't passive. It's not like parking your car in the garage, switching off the lights, and hoping it's still there in the morning. Sleep is more like taking your car into a high-tech auto shop that works on your engine, repaints the bumper, upgrades your tires, and throws in a new transmission for free—all while you're blissfully unaware, dreaming about the time you accidentally called your third-grade teacher "Mom."

Sleep is an active, highly coordinated process your brain and body go through to repair, refresh, and rebuild.

Without it, you're not just tired. You're a mess at the molecular level.

What Happens When You Sleep

When you fall asleep, your brain and body don't just shut down. They shift into a series of carefully orchestrated stages, cycling through different types of sleep over and over through the night. The two big players in this nightly dance are Non-REM sleep and REM sleep.

Non-REM sleep is like the deep-cleaning crew. Early in the night, you drift through light stages of sleep where your muscles relax, your heart rate drops, and your body temperature falls. If someone whispers your name or the cat jumps on your bed, you might wake up easily during this phase. But slip a little deeper, and you enter the heavy-lifting stages: slow-wave sleep.

In slow-wave sleep, your brain waves slow down, your body releases growth hormone, your immune system kicks into high gear, and your brain starts doing something remarkable—taking out the trash. Literally.

Inside your brain, cerebrospinal fluid pulses rhythmically, washing away the metabolic waste that builds up while you're awake. Think of it like a nightly brain bath. Miss enough slow-wave sleep and it's like missing trash day for a month. Everything piles up, stinks to high heaven, and makes it a lot harder to function.

REM sleep, on the other hand, is the theater of your dreams. During REM (Rapid Eye Movement) sleep, your brain lights up like Times Square. Neurons fire rapidly, almost as if you were awake. This is the time for wild, vivid dreams, and behind the curtain, critical work is going on: your brain is consolidating memories, processing emotions, and fine-tuning your cognitive skills. Miss out on REM sleep and it's like trying to run a business while forgetting all your passwords and bursting into tears every time the copier jams.

The Sleep Cycle

A normal sleep cycle takes about 90 minutes, and healthy adults cycle through four to six of these per night. Early in the night, you spend more time in slow-wave sleep. Toward morning, you spend longer stretches in REM. It's like a perfectly timed relay race, with each stage handing the baton off to the next.

The problem arises when this race gets tripped up—by stress, caffeine, blue light, racing thoughts, or even the neighbor's dog who thinks midnight is a fine time for a barking recital. Fragmented sleep means your body never gets the full benefits of each stage, and it shows. You wake up feeling like you've been hit by a truck, even if you technically "slept" for eight hours.

A more effective approach is to focus not just on how much you sleep, but how well you sleep—and that brings us to the quality of sleep, not just the quantity.

What Counts as Good Sleep

Good sleep isn't measured just by the number of hours you spend drooling on your pillow. It's measured by how much restorative sleep you get, how many times you wake up during the night, and how refreshed you feel in the morning.

A healthy adult needs about seven to nine hours of sleep per night. But it's not just about logging hours like you're clocking in for a shift at the factory. It's about how much deep sleep and REM sleep you manage to get during that time. Ideally, about 20–25% of your sleep should be REM, and another 20–25% should be deep, slow-wave sleep.

In measurable terms, good sleep looks like falling asleep within about twenty minutes of hitting the pillow, staying asleep with minimal wake-ups, getting enough deep and REM sleep, and waking up feeling like a halfway functional human instead of a cast member from *The Walking Dead*.

Signs You're Getting Great Sleep

You know you're getting great sleep when you wake up naturally, without an alarm, and you don't feel the immediate urge to trade your soul for five more minutes under the covers. Your mood is stable, your memory sharp, and your body feels capable of handling the random curveballs the day throws at you.

In real life, most of us have a few hiccups here and there. But if you're sleeping well most nights— meaning you fall asleep relatively easily, sleep through the night, and wake up feeling restored—

you're doing better than a large chunk of the population.

Quick story for you: I once hiked 20 miles in a single day along the Michigan Shore to Shore Trail. By the time I set up camp under the stars and zipped into my sleeping bag, I was so wiped out that a raccoon rummaging through my gear didn't even register. I slept like a rock.

When I finally woke up, the sunrise was golden, my body felt rested and my brain was sharp—sharp enough to spot the mess that little visitor had made of my pack. That's what great sleep feels like. You wake up ready for anything, even if the next trail town is suffering from a tragic coffee shortage.

Why Modern Life Wrecks Sleep

If sleep is so vital, why do we treat it like an optional add-on, somewhere between flossing and cleaning out the garage?

The truth is, modern life is designed to mess with our sleep. Screens, noise, stress, weird work schedules, and the omnipresent idea that being busy is a badge of honor all conspire to make sleep harder than it needs to be.

The human body evolved to follow the rhythms of the sun—wake with the light, sleep with the darkness. But now we sit under artificial lights, stare at screens that blast blue light into our brains, drink caffeine until sunset, and wonder why we can't drift off like we did when we were kids.

The solution lies in resetting your relationship with sleep. It's not an interruption to your life. It's the foundation for living well. Great sleep isn't just possible; it's natural—once you understand what your body and mind need to make it happen.

How to Build Better Sleep

Achieving great sleep means giving your body the conditions it needs to cycle naturally through all the stages of sleep, without unnecessary disruptions.

That means sticking to a regular sleep schedule, managing your exposure to light, creating a cool and dark sleep environment, winding down properly before bed, and managing stress during the day. It sounds simple—and it is—but simple doesn't mean easy. The real work lies in making small, consistent choices that add up over time.

One of my favorite examples comes from a friend of mine who used to be a night owl. He would stay up late, scrolling, gaming, you name it. Then he would drag himself through the next day like a zombie. He finally committed to a simple, regular bedtime routine: shutting off screens an hour before bed, lowering the lights, and reading a paperback instead of staring at his phone. Within a month, he wasn't just sleeping better—he was sharper, happier, and had energy to spare. His only complaint? He wished he had done it ten years earlier.

Sleep Debt and Recovery

Some people think they can cheat sleep during the week and make up for it on the weekends. While there's some truth to the idea that you can recover a little from short-term sleep deprivation, it's not a winning long-term strategy.

Chronic sleep debt changes the way your body regulates hormones, processes sugar, manages appetite, and even fights off disease.

The real fix is consistency. Aim to give yourself enough opportunity for sleep every night—not just when it's convenient. Sleep isn't a luxury. It's the factory reset your body needs to stay sane, healthy, and alive.

Sleep Is Your Secret Weapon

Sleep isn't an interruption to your life; it's the very thing that gives you the energy, clarity, and resilience to live your life fully. It's not a chore. It's a gift.

By understanding what sleep really is, appreciating the stages your body needs to cycle through, and valuing the quality of your sleep as much as the quantity, you can start to see sleep not as passive downtime but as the ultimate act of self-care and restoration.

Getting great sleep is not a pipe dream. It's a reality waiting for you—one night, one habit, one good choice at a time.

As you move through the rest of this book, you'll find simple strategies, smarter routines, and a few mindset shifts that can help you take back your sleep —and with it, the superpower you were always meant to wield.

But before we get too serious, let's take a quick detour into the wild, weird, and sometimes downright hilarious ways people have tried to catch some shut-eye over the centuries. Trust me, it'll make you appreciate your boring old pillow a whole lot more.

The Most Bizarre, Hilarious, and Fascinating Sleep Remedies Ever Devised

"Humans: inventors of fire, flight, and vibrating sleep goggles." — Rogue Librarian Wisdom

There were several things I discovered about sleep in my research. Every living creature with a brain needs rest, yet humans have spent centuries concocting increasingly ludicrous ways to accomplish something that dogs, cats, and even sloths seem to master effortlessly. While other species curl up and drift off without an existential crisis, people have employed everything from narcotic elixirs to vibrating sleep goggles. Some of these remedies come from ancient civilizations, while others have been born from modern desperation, but they all share one thing in common: sheer absurdity.

Sleep Temples, Hammocks, and the Delusions of Ancient Insomniacs

The ancient Egyptians, who gave the world the pyramids and hieroglyphics, also pioneered the idea of sleep temples. These were not casual napping spots but elaborate institutions where priests performed rituals, chanted mystical phrases, and encouraged desperate insomniacs to seek divine intervention. Rather than simply shutting their eyes and letting exhaustion do its job, people traveled great distances to lie on sacred stone slabs and wait for a god to take pity on them.

This method is no longer recommended, not only because it lacks scientific backing but because getting to a sleep temple in today's world would require multiple layovers and an uncomfortable seat in economy class, which are the exact opposite of sleep-inducing experiences.

Hammocks, on the other hand, have remained a staple of relaxation across cultures. The Mayans and other indigenous groups figured out early that gently rocking back and forth could lull a person to sleep, much like a well-secured baby in a cradle. Modern science supports this, showing that rocking can synchronize brain waves and promote deeper sleep.

However, practical issues abound. Not everyone has the coordination to gracefully enter a hammock. Those who do often find themselves waking up in an undignified heap of tangled blankets on the floor.

The Endless Parade of Gadgets and Gimmicks

People will buy anything if it promises to fix their problems without requiring effort. This is why the sleep industry has spawned an entire market of bizarre gadgets. One particularly ambitious invention is the Somnox Sleep Robot, a soft, oblong pillow that mimics breathing patterns to lull its user into slumber. It's like spooning a small, overpriced lap pillow, minus the emotional baggage of a real relationship.

For those who enjoy feeling like they're starring in a low-budget sci-fi experiment, there are vibrating sleep goggles that claim to massage away stress and lull your face into dreamland. These gadgets often combine gentle vibration, heat, and even soft music or white noise to help relax the facial muscles and promote calm. Some models look like something you'd wear to pilot a spaceship—bonus points if you enjoy confusing your spouse or terrifying the dog.

But do they work? Well, *maybe*. While there isn't a mountain of peer-reviewed research backing these devices, there is some logic to the method. Gentle massage and warmth around the eyes can stimulate the parasympathetic nervous system—the part of your brain that says, "Let's slow things down." For some people, that's just enough to shift from racing thoughts to restful drowsiness.

If you're going to try one, opt for a model with adjustable heat, soft padding, and a timer function. Look for rechargeable options with good reviews and skip the ones that sound like a jackhammer when they vibrate (because, obviously). And like any sleep aid, these goggles should complement a good routine—not replace one. If your bedroom still feels like a lava pit or you're mainlining energy drinks at 4 p.m., not even the fanciest face gadget is going to save you.

Still, if you're curious—and open to looking a little ridiculous—it might be worth experimenting with one of these high-tech sleep masks. Just don't forget to take it off before your morning Zoom call.

Perfumed pajamas are another modern oddity, based on the idea that smelling like lavender will trick the brain into thinking it's time to rest. Scent-based relaxation is nothing new—ancient Romans used herbal infusions to calm the nerves—but the idea of specifically infusing sleepwear with fragrance feels like a marketing department's fever dream. Lavender may be soothing, but no amount of perfumed fabric can undo the damage of an ill-timed espresso.

Liquid Courage and the Questionable Role of Alcohol in Sleep

For centuries, people have turned to alcohol to speed up the journey to unconsciousness. A stiff drink has long been a go-to sleep aid, with everyone from medieval monks to overworked parents. While alcohol does have sedative effects, it also ensures that sleep will be fragmented. Those who pass out quickly from a few too many glasses of wine often wake up at 3 AM.

Modern variations of this trend include sleep-inducing mocktails, which promise all the relaxation without the hangover. These concoctions often contain magnesium, melatonin, or chamomile, and they might help—but only if the person drinking them is already prepared to wind down. No beverage, no matter how soothing, can counteract scrolling through the news.

Counting Sheep, Cognitive Shuffling, and Other Mind Games

Counting sheep is the most famous sleep remedy, mostly because it's easy to visualize and requires no equipment. The idea is that monotonous mental activity will lull the brain into submission. However, not everyone finds this effective. Some people get too caught up in sheep logistics, wondering if they are all the same breed, where they are jumping from, and if someone is responsible for rounding them up afterward. This is not a restful train of thought.

A more modern variation, the cognitive shuffle, involves thinking of random, unrelated words to prevent overthinking. This technique attempts to distract the brain from stressors, which sounds promising until the chosen words are too interesting. One moment, someone is thinking about "banana," "cloud," and "marshmallow," and the next, they are pondering the history of aviation or debating whether bananas are technically berries. The technique might work for some, but for overactive thinkers, it's a gateway to another sleepless night.

Cognitive Behavioral Therapy for Insomnia (CBT-I) is another science-backed approach that helps rewire the thoughts and habits that keep you awake. Studies show it can be more effective than medication for chronic sleep issues. Instead of popping a pill, you retrain your brain to stop treating bedtime like a battle.

CBT-I targets the unhelpful thought patterns and behaviors that quietly sabotage your sleep. You know, those internal monologues that kick in the moment your head hits the pillow: *"If I fall asleep right now, I'll get six hours. Wait, now it's five hours. What if I'm awake all night again? I'll be useless tomorrow. Why can't I just sleep like a normal human being?"* CBT-I helps you stop that spiral before it pulls you into another restless night.

And this isn't just feel-good psychology—it works. Numerous studies (including those cited by the American College of Physicians and the NIH) show that CBT-I is often more effective than sleep medication for chronic insomnia, with longer-lasting results and no groggy side effects. In fact, it's now considered the *first-line treatment* for insomnia, meaning it's the gold standard—not a last resort.

So how does it work? It typically involves a structured program over several weeks, often with the help of a trained therapist or a digital platform. You learn how to identify and challenge anxious sleep thoughts, set a consistent sleep schedule, improve sleep efficiency, and gradually retrain your brain to associate your bed with sleeping—not tossing, turning, or mentally drafting your grocery list at 1:30 a.m.

For those not ready to see a therapist in person (or just not thrilled about explaining their bedtime routine to a stranger), there are excellent online programs and apps like Somryst, Sleepio, or CBT-I Coach—each offering guided lessons, tracking tools, and exercises to build better habits.

If you've tried everything else and still find yourself losing the battle at bedtime, CBT-I might be your next best step. It's not magic, and it's not always quick—but it works. Because sometimes, the most powerful thing

you can do for your sleep isn't buying another gadget or googling "why am I still awake?" for the thousandth time... it's changing the way you think about sleep in the first place.

The Internet's Contribution to Sleep Deprivation

In the grand tradition of making everything weird, the internet has introduced a new breed of sleep aids. ASMR (Autonomous Sensory Meridian Response) videos feature people whispering, tapping, or performing mundane tasks in hushed tones, allegedly triggering a relaxation response. For some, these videos induce deep calm; for others, they are profoundly unsettling, like eavesdropping on an overly intimate phone call.

Sleep podcasts take a similar approach. "Sleep With Me," hosted by Drew Ackerman, is intentionally designed to be boring. He rambles in a droning monotone, covering topics so mundane that the brain gives up and shuts down. It's a brilliant concept, though it does raise questions about how one's life has unraveled to the point where they willingly listen to someone explain the organizational structure of a spice rack at bedtime.

Perhaps the strangest internet-era sleep trend is the rise of sleep livestreams. On platforms like Twitch, people literally film themselves sleeping while thousands of viewers tune in. Some streamers even allow audience members to donate money to trigger noises, flashing lights, or other disruptions. This is less of a sleep aid and more of a performance art piece, proving once again that the internet will turn anything into entertainment, even unconsciousness.

What This All Means for Actual Sleep

The history of sleep remedies is a testament to human ingenuity, desperation, and an unwavering belief that the right trick will finally unlock the secret to rest. Some methods, like hammocks and controlled breathing, have scientific merit. Others, like vibrating goggles and whisper-induced relaxation, depend entirely on personal preference. What remains true is that sleep cannot be forced. Chasing sleep too aggressively only makes it more elusive, much like trying to grab a cloud or reason with a toddler.

There is no single magic cure, but there is humor in the attempt. Anyone who has ever tried a ridiculous sleep hack—whether it was chugging warm milk, listening to a podcast about shoelaces, or cuddling a robotic breathing pillow—can at least take comfort in the fact that they are not alone.

Humanity has been fighting this battle for centuries, and if history is any indication, we will continue inventing absurd solutions for the simplest biological function until the end of time.

Humans have tried just about everything to catch some Z's—some methods more questionable (and hilarious) than others. But before you start stuffing your pillow with lettuce or chanting to the moon, there's one modern sleep aid that's actually worth a closer look. It's called melatonin, and unlike some of the bizarre rituals we just covered, this one's got a little more real science behind it.

Let's dive into what it is, how it works, and why popping a melatonin gummy might just beat rubbing slug slime on your forehead.

Melatonin: The Sandman's Little Helper or Just Another Sleepy Time Myth?

"Melatonin: because nothing says 'natural sleep' like a pill from aisle five." — Anonymous

You've seen it sitting there in the vitamin aisle, right between the fish oil and the multivitamins, promising the kind of deep, effortless sleep usually reserved for hibernating bears. "Take me," it whispers, "and you'll drift off in no time." But before you pop that little pill and expect the Sandman to personally escort you to dreamland, let's take a closer look. Does melatonin really help you sleep better, or is it just another supplement?

The Good: Does Melatonin Work?

Science gives us a cautiously optimistic nod. A meta-analysis—(Quick side note. And yes, calling it a "side note" is a bit of a misnomer, because this detour is going to park itself squarely in the middle of the text.)

When I first heard the term meta-analysis, I assumed it had something to do with a Jedi-level power of analysis—maybe a superhuman ability to see through the noise and pull truth from the swirling data void.

Naturally, in my training as a librarian superhero (cape optional, reading glasses mandatory), I was excited. "Ah," I thought, "this is where the wise ones dwell." Turns out, it's more like the academic version of rummaging through a hundred junk drawers to find one matching spoon.

A meta-analysis, for the uninitiated, is when researchers take a pile of individual studies on a specific topic—say, the impact of blue light on sleep, or whether the temperature in your bedroom has any effect on your circadian rhythm—and smoosh all the results together to look for patterns. They don't gather fresh data; they let others do the heavy lifting, then crunch all those findings into one super-sized, spreadsheet-laden stew. Ideally, this creates a clearer picture. In practice? Sometimes it's more like stirring glitter into soup and calling it clarity.

Here's what really blew my Dewey-decimal-organized mind: you can find meta-analyses supporting *either* side of almost any sleep issue. One meta-analysis swears naps are the secret to productivity; another insists they are the gateway drug to a lifetime of insomnia. Depends which one you read.

Makes you think. Not necessarily sleep, but definitely think. So yes, it's a rabbit trail—but hopefully one that leaves you just a little more skeptical, a little more curious, and a lot less impressed the next time someone says, "According to a meta-analysis…"

Now, back to the meta-analysis on melatonin.

As I was saying, science gives us a cautiously optimistic nod. According to a 2013 meta-analysis published in *PLoS ONE,* a meta-analysis—found that melatonin can reduce the time it takes to fall asleep by about seven minutes and slightly extend total sleep time. Not exactly a knockout punch, but if you're the kind of person who counts every extra minute of shuteye as a victory, it might be worth considering. Some research suggests it's particularly effective for those with delayed sleep phase syndrome—people whose bodies naturally want to stay up late and sleep in. If you've ever found yourself wide awake at 2 a.m. but groggy and dysfunctional at 7 a.m., melatonin might help realign your internal clock.

The Not-So-Good: Side Effects and Limitations

Now, before you start treating melatonin like a nightly ritual, let's talk about the fine print. Some people report grogginess the next day, almost like a hangover without the fun memories. Others experience vivid dreams, nausea, dizziness, or headaches.

More concerning is that melatonin doesn't work for everyone, and it's not a magic fix for chronic insomnia. Sleep experts emphasize that melatonin is more effective for shifting sleep schedules—like adjusting to jet lag or an early morning shift—than for curing general sleeplessness. Overuse can also mess with your natural melatonin production, meaning your body might become dependent on an outside source instead of making its own sleep magic.

To Melatonin or Not to Melatonin (That Is the Sleepy Question)

Melatonin has its place—long distance jet travel, night shifts, or when your internal clock thinks it lives in another time zone. But let's not kid ourselves: if you're dealing with chronic insomnia, a supplement won't fix

what a solid bedtime routine can. And honestly, no pill can replace the simple, underrated power of respecting your body's need for rest.

Because here's the deal: even the best sleep aid can't outwork bad habits. As you will see in the coming chapters, if your nighttime routine involves blue-lit screens, erratic bedtimes, or cheeseburgers at midnight, you're not setting yourself up for slumber success. You're setting the stage for a 2 a.m. staring contest with the ceiling.

In the next chapter, we'll crack open the medicine cabinet and peek into the world of modern sleep solutions. Some are promising. Some are…well, you'll see.

Cutting Edge Pharmacological Sleep Solutions: Beyond Counting Sheep

"There is no medicine like hope… and maybe a decent mattress." — Orison Swett Marden (adapted)

In the quest for better sleep, modern medicine has gone far beyond warm milk and bedtime stories. The pharmaceutical industry has developed a range of medications designed to help people fall asleep faster, stay asleep longer, and wake up feeling more refreshed. But not all sleep aids are created equal, and some come with side effects that make them more trouble than they're worth.

Fortunately, recent advances have led to new medications that work differently than the traditional sleep drugs of the past.

One of the biggest breakthroughs is a class of drugs called Dual Orexin Receptor Antagonists, or DORAs. Unlike older medications that sedate the entire brain, these target the orexin system—the part responsible for keeping you awake. By blocking orexin, they essentially turn down the body's "wakefulness switch," helping people drift off without the grogginess or risk of dependence older sleep aids can cause.

The first of these, suvorexant (Belsomra), helps people fall asleep faster and stay asleep longer, though some users report morning grogginess, especially at higher doses. Other DORAs, such as lemborexant (Dayvigo) and daridorexant (Quviviq), have followed, with daridorexant standing out for reducing next-day fatigue.

Researchers are also working on a more refined version called Selective Orexin Receptor Antagonists (SORAs). These block only one of the two orexin receptors, aiming for the same benefits with even fewer side effects. Seltorexant, one promising candidate, is still in trials but shows early signs of helping people fall asleep without heavy next-day drowsiness.

For decades, the go-to sleep meds were benzodiazepines and their cousins, the "Z-drugs." Benzodiazepines like temazepam and lorazepam enhance GABA, a neurotransmitter that slows brain activity and sedates. Effective short-term? Yes. But they come with a high risk of dependence and ugly withdrawal symptoms if used long-term.

Z-drugs, like zolpidem (Ambien) and eszopiclone (Lunesta), were developed as a safer alternative. They work similarly on GABA receptors and are less likely to cause dependence—but not without quirks, like strange sleep behaviors (think sleepwalking or even sleep-driving) that have raised safety concerns.

Some doctors also prescribe sedating antidepressants like trazodone or doxepin for people juggling both depression and insomnia. They can help, but often bring next-day drowsiness and unwanted weight gain.

Newer experimental drugs like vornorexant aim to improve sleep while reducing grogginess, but more research is needed before they hit the shelves.

While prescription sleep aids can be helpful, they aren't magic bullets. They work best when paired with solid sleep habits: a regular sleep schedule, less screen time before bed, and a relaxing bedtime routine.

Many specialists recommend Cognitive Behavioral Therapy for Insomnia (CBT-I) as a first-line treatment before medication. Studies show CBT-I can effectively retrain your brain for better sleep without the side effects that pills sometimes bring.

As research continues, the future of sleep medicine looks promising: faster sleep onset, better rest, fewer side effects. But no matter how fancy the meds get, the foundation of good sleep will always come down to how we treat our bodies, our minds, and our daily routines.

Now, before we leave the world of pharmacological sleep solutions, I feel obligated—if not morally, then at least genetically—to disclose something here: my dad was a pharmacist. Not just the kind behind the counter, but the real deal—he had a doctorate in pharmacology and taught pharmacy at the university level for twenty seven years. He always hoped I'd follow in his footsteps, and carry the family banner into the world of compounding, counting by fives and using very tiny measuring spoons.

That dream lasted until the day I sat in a college chemistry lab, blankly staring at a beaker while my lab partner joyfully mashed, mixed, and measured like some caffeinated apothecary. Everyone seemed to know exactly what they were doing. I, however, was mostly trying not to light anything on fire. Right then and there, I realized two things: one, I had absolutely no idea what the experiment was, and two, I'd be much happier in a literature class reading about fictional disasters instead of causing real ones in a lab. I dropped the class and happily enrolled in another English course. No regrets.

My brother Brian, on the other hand, did carry the torch and became a retail pharmacist. He gets to use long, unpronounceable drug names with confidence and correct my pronunciation at family dinners. And yet here I am, writing a chapter about the pharmacology of sleep, holding my own with the terminology—even if I say half of it like I'm auditioning for a foreign film. Somewhere, I think our dad is proud. Or at least chuckling. Probably both.

Since we're already talking about the go-to fixes people reach for when sleep goes sideways, let's shift from pills to pixels. Because if there's one thing modern life has taught us, there's probably a gadget for that. So what exactly is the world of sleep tech promising these days? Smarter beds? Dream-detecting headbands? A wearable that whispers lullabies into your wrist?Let's find out. The future of sleep might just come with a charging cable.

The Digital Insomniac's Dilemma

"Technology: helping you lose sleep since the invention of the lightbulb." — Anonymous

Technology, as a concept, was supposed to make our lives easier. Somewhere along the way, it decided to hijack our sleep instead. At first, it was subtle. The electric light extended our days beyond sunset, and televisions crept into bedrooms under the guise of relaxation.

Then came computers, smartphones, and social media, each progressively more adept at keeping us awake for reasons that, in the cold light of morning, seem ridiculous. If you've ever sacrificed sleep to watch a video titled *Ten Ways Squirrels Are Secretly Planning World Domination*, you already understand how easily technology can derail an evening.

At its core, technology is neither good nor bad. It simply follows human nature, amplifying whatever impulses we feed it. The problem is that modern tech is designed to hold our attention, and sleep, unfortunately, is the moment we relinquish it entirely. From blue light exposure to endless scrolling, the very tools meant to improve our lives have become some of the biggest obstacles to restful sleep.

Sleep Technology: Promise vs. Reality

Not all technology is out to ruin sleep. A growing industry is devoted to fixing the very problem it helped create. Sleep trackers, white noise machines, smart mattresses, and blue light filtering glasses have all entered the market, promising to restore rest to a sleepless world. Some of these technologies show promise, particularly those that enhance sleep hygiene rather than disrupt it.

Wearable devices, for example, provide valuable insights into sleep patterns. Fitness trackers and smartwatches monitor heart rate variability, movement, and breathing to estimate sleep cycles. While not 100% accurate, they can reveal general trends, like whether you're getting enough deep sleep or if your so-called "eight hours" includes two hours of tossing and turning.

The flaw is that these devices can sometimes make people obsess over sleep data, creating stress about the very thing they are trying to improve. Sleep performance anxiety—yes, that's a real thing—can make people so preoccupied with their sleep scores that they actually sleep worse.

Then there are smart mattresses, capable of adjusting firmness based on body position and even regulating temperature. This would be ideal if all sleep problems were mechanical in nature. But even a perfectly optimized bed won't help if the real issue is anxiety, poor sleep habits, or an ill-advised espresso at 9 p.m.

The Real Problem With Technology and Sleep

The biggest offender in the tech-sleep war is the screen. Tablets, phones, and laptops emit blue light, which suppresses melatonin, the hormone that signals to the body that it's time to sleep. Exposure to this light tricks the brain into thinking it's still daytime, delaying the natural sleep process.

Most people are aware of this by now, yet the nightly scrolling continues. The problem isn't just the blue light. It's the engagement. Checking an email "one last time" might result in a 30-minute spiral. Social media, designed to provoke emotion, can trigger everything from political rage to an existential crisis over a former classmate's suspiciously perfect vacation photos. Even reading a stimulating e-book can keep the brain wired instead of winding down.

A Smarter Approach to Sleep Tech

Fighting technology with more technology sounds counterintuitive, but in the right hands, it works. The key is using tech in ways that support, rather than sabotage, the sleep process.

The simplest, most effective change is to control light exposure. Blue light blocking glasses can help, but they're not a free pass for scrolling through news headlines at midnight. A better solution is to dim screens well before bedtime. Many devices now offer "night mode," which reduces blue light emission. However, this is only part of the equation. The real issue is not the light itself but what's happening on the screen. The goal should be to limit engagement with content that stimulates the brain.

A more structured approach involves setting clear boundaries with devices. This includes establishing a "tech curfew," a specific time when screens go off for the night. Ideally, this happens at least an hour before bed. This isn't about deprivation—it's about reclaiming the ability to wind down naturally. Replacing screen time with low-tech alternatives—

reading a physical book, journaling, or listening to calming music—helps retrain the brain to expect sleep at a consistent time.

Avoiding Common Pitfalls

One common mistake people make when adopting sleep technology is relying too heavily on data without considering personal experience. If a sleep tracker claims you had a terrible night, but you feel rested, trust your body over the algorithm. Conversely, if the tracker shows perfect sleep but you feel exhausted, don't dismiss your own experience. Technology is a tool, not a judge.

Another issue is overcomplicating the sleep process. It's tempting to load up on every gadget available, from white noise machines to weighted blankets to smart alarms that wake you during the "optimal" sleep stage. While some of these tools are helpful, adding too many can create stress rather than relief. Sleep isn't something that needs to be micromanaged—it's something that needs to be allowed.

An Exercise in Disconnection

To truly understand how technology affects your sleep, it helps to experiment. Choose one night to go completely tech-free for an hour before bed. No phones, no tablets, no TV. Instead, opt for something analog—a book, a conversation, or simply sitting in silence. Notice how your body responds. If sleep comes more easily, it's a sign that technology has been interfering more than you realized.

For those who rely on screens for winding down, a compromise might be needed. Audiobooks or podcasts with calm narration can provide entertainment without the visual stimulation. Smart lighting systems that gradually dim can help signal to the brain that it's time to sleep, mimicking the natural sunset. The key is intentionality—using technology as a support system, not a crutch.

Final Thoughts On Tech

Technology isn't the enemy, but it definitely needs a leash. The best sleep solutions come from balancing its perks with the realities of human biology. Sleep isn't some glitch you fix with another gadget; it's a process you nurture with better habits.

The real challenge isn't finding the right tools—it's remembering to use them like a human, not a lab rat. If you're navigating the shiny, blinking world of sleep tech, remember the most important rule:

control your technology before it controls you. The night belongs to rest, not notifications, not step counters, and definitely not a mattress that emails you about your tossing and turning.

Now, speaking of nights gone wrong…

Let's talk about insomnia—the ancient, stubborn, maddening beast that no gadget can tame. (Spoiler alert: you can.)

The Truth About Insomnia (And Why You Can Fix It)

"Insomnia is a gross feeder. It will nourish itself on any kind of thinking, including thinking about not thinking." — Clifton Fadiman

Harold had a gift. Not a useful one like juggling or speaking five languages—no, his gift was lying awake at night for hours, thinking about ridiculous things. Like, why do we say "slept like a baby" when babies wake up screaming every two hours? Or, if he were stranded on a desert island, would he rather have unlimited tacos or an endless supply of coffee? The more exhausted he got, the weirder the thoughts became. Meanwhile, sleep? Nowhere to be found.

He tried everything. Flipping the pillow to the cool side, rearranging his blankets with the precision of a NASA engineer, even performing the ancient ritual of "staring at the ceiling and counting the sheep as they waddled by." Nothing worked. So he checked the clock. Did the math. Groaned. Realized he was down to just a few hours of potential sleep—if only his brain would cooperate. And thus, the night continued in an endless loop of frustration, until sheer exhaustion finally took over. By morning, he woke up groggy, annoyed, and already dreading another night of the same nonsense.

Determined to fix it, he went all in. Melatonin, sleep teas, eye masks, expensive pillows, lavender-scented sprays—if someone on the internet claimed it helped with sleep, Harold tried it. When none of it worked, he resigned himself to the idea that he was just "one of those people" who couldn't sleep. He started saying things like "I've always been a night owl" and "My brain just doesn't shut off," fully accepting his new identity as a caffeine-dependent insomniac.

But here's the truth: insomnia is not a personality trait. It's not a lifelong curse. It's simply a malfunction of a process the body already knows how to do. The problem isn't that sleep is broken—it's that something is disrupting it. Fixing sleep isn't about hunting down the perfect pillow or discovering some mystical supplement. It's about removing the barriers keeping the body from doing what it's designed to do. And the good news? That's entirely possible.

The Flaws in the Most Common Sleep Advice

Most sleep advice falls into two categories: quick fixes and vague instructions.

The quick fixes are things like melatonin, sleep aids, and herbal remedies. They might work short-term, but they don't solve the real problem. Melatonin can help with jet lag, but it's not a cure for chronic insomnia. Sleep medications can knock you out, but they don't create natural, restorative sleep.

None of these things address why sleep isn't happening in the first place.

Then there's the vague advice: "Relax." "Don't stress about it." "Just go to bed earlier." These suggestions aren't just unhelpful—they're actively frustrating. Telling someone with insomnia to relax is like telling someone in a sinking boat to stop worrying about the water.

And the idea that people just need to go to bed earlier completely ignores the reality of circadian rhythms and sleep pressure.

Another common myth? That everyone needs exactly eight hours of sleep. It's been drilled into our heads like a universal law.

The truth is, sleep needs vary. Some people thrive on six and a half hours, while others need nine. What matters more than the number is the quality of your sleep.

Someone who gets eight hours of restless, interrupted sleep will feel worse than someone who gets six hours of deep, uninterrupted rest.

A Better Approach to Fixing Sleep

Restoring natural sleep starts with understanding that it's a full-day process. The choices you make in the morning, afternoon, and evening all contribute to what happens at night.

Sleep doesn't begin when you get into bed—it begins the moment you wake up.The first step is resetting your internal clock. Your brain relies on light to regulate the sleep-wake cycle.

When you don't get enough bright light in the morning and get too much artificial light at night, your circadian rhythm gets thrown off.

The simplest fix? Get outside for at least twenty minutes in the morning. Dim the lights in the evening. And put away the screens an hour before bed to prevent blue light from messing with your melatonin.

The second step is establishing a consistent sleep schedule. Your body loves routine. Going to bed and waking up at the same time every day—even on weekends—strengthens your natural sleep cycle.

Sleeping in on weekends might feel good, but it confuses your internal clock and makes Sunday nights miserable.

The third step is fixing your bedtime routine. Many people expect their brains to go from fully alert to sound asleep like flipping a switch. That's not how sleep works. Your body needs a transition period.

A simple pre-bed routine—reading, stretching, or listening to calming music—signals to your brain that sleep is coming.

Consistency is key. Doing the same wind-down activities every night trains your brain to associate them with sleep.

The Mistakes That Keep People Stuck

The biggest mistake people make is changing too much at once. They overhaul their entire routine overnight—cutting caffeine, eliminating screens, meditating, taking supplements, implementing a two-hour wind-down... all in one go.

It's overwhelming. And it rarely sticks.

Small, consistent changes work better than massive overhauls.

Another mistake? Only focusing on nighttime habits. Sleep is affected by everything—meal timing, stress levels, light exposure.

Eat a heavy meal right before bed, slam coffee at 4 PM, sit under fluorescent lights all day—and you've stacked the odds against yourself long before your head hits the pillow.

Finally, many people assume that if they don't fall asleep immediately, they've failed. This creates a nasty cycle of frustration and anxiety that makes sleep even harder. Sleep isn't instant. Allowing time to relax—without putting pressure on the process— is essential.

A Simple Change to Try Tonight

Start small. Before bed, take five minutes to write down everything that's on your mind. This clears mental clutter and separates thinking time from sleeping time.

Keep a small notebook by the bed. If you're lying awake, instead of stewing about it, write down what's keeping you up. This simple habit retrains your brain to offload worries onto paper instead of carrying them into sleep.

(If you happen to be a writer, this is also a sneaky way to gather future book ideas.)

Reframing Sleep as a Natural Process

Insomnia isn't a life sentence. It's a system that needs a reset. Instead of chasing quick fixes, focusing on the full-day approach to sleep leads to lasting change.

Understanding why insomnia happens—and how small, simple adjustments can fix it—is the first step. The most important shift right now? Sleep isn't something you fight for. It's something you allow.

In the next chapter, we'll get into what I consider my number one piece of advice—the go-to strategy I recommend when people are completely fed up and just want someone to tell them *what to do*.

Remember that chapter on sleep triage? When things are really falling apart, this is one of the two chapters I send people to first. If you're still looking for the "just give it to me straight" plan, don't go anywhere. This is it.

Earn Your Sleep: Move More

"Sleep like a baby? First, tire yourself out like a toddler at a theme park." — Unknown

Last weekend, I was at a wedding reception, making small talk between bites of steak crostini, when someone asked about my latest book. I told them it was about sleep. They leaned in and said, "Alright, then—what's the single best piece of advice you can give me?" I thought about it for a second, ran through all the research, my own experiences, and the countless sleep struggles I've heard about. Then I said, "Get physically tired. Go move. Exercise. Do something that makes your body ready for rest."

I realized that the best nights of sleep I've ever had weren't because of a fancy pillow or some mystical bedtime routine. They happened after long days of hiking, grueling two-a-day practices, or just a day filled with good, hard work. When my body was truly tired, sleep wasn't a struggle—it was inevitable.

And that's the first, simplest thing I'd tell anyone struggling with sleep: Make your body so ready for rest that it can't argue with you when you lie down at night.

The connection between physical activity and sleep quality is undeniable. The body is designed to move, and when it doesn't, it rebels. Sleep struggles are often the body's way of saying, "You haven't earned your rest." In a world where sitting is the default—commuting, working, unwinding in front of screens —it's no wonder so many people struggle to sleep. Movement is the missing ingredient, the foundational element that sets the stage for deep, restorative rest.

The Body in Motion, the Mind at Rest

Sleep isn't just about shutting down—it's about recovery. And nothing creates a need for recovery quite like movement. Research shows that people who engage in regular physical activity fall asleep faster, wake up less frequently, and enjoy deeper, more restorative sleep. Exercise doesn't just burn energy; it resets the entire system. It regulates body temperature, stabilizes hormones, and quiets the nervous system—all of which make sleep come easier. But not all movement is created equal when it comes to sleep. The best approach combines aerobic activity, resistance training, and relaxation-based practices to prepare both the body and mind for rest.

Movement that Matters

Aerobic Exercise: Resetting the Sleep-Wake Cycle

Walking, jogging, cycling—these forms of cardio work wonders for sleep. Regular aerobic activity strengthens the body's circadian rhythm, reinforcing the natural signals that distinguish day from night. Even just 30 minutes of moderate-intensity movement most days of the week can make a huge difference in falling asleep and staying asleep.

Strength Training: Deeper Sleep Through Recovery

Resistance training—whether with body weight or weights—promotes deeper sleep cycles. Muscles require repair, and that repair happens during the deepest stages of sleep. People who strength train consistently tend to experience fewer nighttime awakenings and a greater percentage of slow-wave sleep, the most restorative phase of the sleep cycle.

Mind-Body Practices: The Transition to Rest

Yoga, tai chi, and stretching routines engage the parasympathetic nervous system, sending signals to the body that it's time to slow down. These exercises, especially when done in the evening, help lower cortisol levels and promote relaxation. A short stretching or yoga session before bed can make the transition to sleep effortless.

Timing Matters

When to exercise? The answer depends on the individual. Morning workouts reinforce circadian rhythms and provide an energy boost for the day. Midday movement prevents the buildup of stress and tension. Evening workouts, if kept moderate, can actually improve sleep—just avoid intense activity within an hour or two of bedtime.

The one thing that doesn't work? Inconsistency. Exercise needs to be a regular part of life, not an occasional burst of effort. The best sleep results come from movement that becomes a daily habit.

Practical Integration: Making Movement Non-Negotiable

For many, the challenge isn't knowing that exercise helps sleep—it's finding the time for it. The key is making movement part of the daily routine. Instead of seeing exercise as another task to squeeze in, look for opportunities to integrate it naturally:

- Walk during phone calls or meetings.

- Take the stairs instead of the elevator.

- Stretch before bed instead of scrolling through your phone.

- Turn household chores into a mini-workout —vacuuming, carrying groceries, even gardening all count as movement.

The biggest mistake? Overcomplicating it. You don't need a gym membership, expensive equipment, or a rigid schedule. The best exercise is the one you'll actually do. Find something enjoyable—hiking, dancing, swimming, playing with the kids—and make it a priority.

Try This Today

Want to see how exercise and movement impacts your sleep? Here's a simple challenge:

Move for at least 30 minutes today. Take a walk, ride a bike, do bodyweight exercises—anything that gets you moving. Then, pay attention to your sleep tonight. Do you fall asleep faster? Sleep more deeply? Feel more refreshed in the morning?

Try it for a few days, and you'll likely notice sleep isn't something you chase. It's something you prepare for. And the best preparation begins with movement.

But movement isn't the only natural way to prepare your body for better sleep.

It turns out there's another kind of workout that's even more relaxing—and you don't even have to leave the bedroom to do it.

Bedroom Benefits: How Sex and Sleep Are Secretly Best Friends

"Sex is like pizza. Even when it's bad, it's still pretty good—and it usually makes you sleepy."
— *Anonymous, but widely attributed to multiple comedians*

L et's go ahead and admit it: you skipped ahead to this chapter, didn't you? And who could blame you?

If every chapter in this book had a homework assignment at the end, this one would get turned in early—and with extra credit.

The Hidden Connection Between Intimacy and Sleep

Now, if you've ever found yourself drifting into sleep after intimacy—or lying there wondering why your partner has already entered REM while you're still wide awake—you've felt the intersection between these two powerhouses of human experience. Let's take a closer look at what's really going on.

What Happens in Your Body After Sex

Sex isn't just a physical activity. It's a full-body, full-brain event that sets off a chain reaction of hormonal shifts, most of which seem tailor-made to help you relax. After climax, your body releases oxytocin, the hormone most responsible for bonding, trust, and feeling like the world is okay again. Alongside that comes prolactin, which is heavily associated with the feeling of post-orgasmic contentment and drowsiness. Dopamine, the feel-good chemical that buzzes during arousal, drops off after orgasm, leaving behind a wave of calm. And cortisol—the stress hormone that does its best to ruin your sleep—takes a significant nosedive.

This is not just poetic theorizing. A 2019 study published in *Frontiers in Public Health* found that sexual activity prior to sleep, especially when it included orgasm, helped people fall asleep faster and stay asleep longer. In short, your body has built-in sleep tech, and it doesn't require a subscription.

Why He's Snoring and You're Still Awake

Of course, not everyone reacts the same way. There's a long-standing joke that men tend to fall asleep immediately afterward while their partners lie awake wondering what just happened. There's a biological reason for that. Research shows that men typically experience a larger surge of prolactin after orgasm than women, which can make sleep arrive faster and hit harder. Women do produce prolactin as well, but the hormonal interplay tends to vary more, often influenced by emotional factors and satisfaction levels. Simply put, if one person is snoring while the other is staring at the ceiling, it's biology talking, not bad manners.

The Two-Way Street Between Sleep and Sex

The relationship between sleep and intimacy runs in both directions. Just as good sex can help you sleep better, good sleep can help you enjoy intimacy more. Lack of quality sleep wreaks havoc on libido. In men, it lowers testosterone, a key driver of desire and performance. In women, it's linked to reduced arousal, more mood swings, and less interest in intimacy overall. One study published in *Sleep Medicine* showed that even a single extra hour of sleep increased sexual desire in women by 14 percent (Kalmbach et al., 2015). Getting more and better sleep is one of the easiest ways to improve both your energy and your connection with the people you care about.

The Power of Physical Affection

It's worth mentioning that physical intimacy doesn't always have to mean sex. Cuddling, touching, and simply lying close to someone you trust can lower cortisol and boost oxytocin, creating the same biological environment that prepares your body for deep, restorative sleep. In fact, a review from the Touch Research Institute found that physical affection before bed led to fewer nighttime awakenings and longer periods of deep sleep (Field, 2010).

Why Connection Matters More Than Performance

Still, not every encounter guarantees a trip to dreamland. If your experience is stressful, disconnected, or emotionally painful, the opposite can happen. In those cases, cortisol levels can spike and anxiety can climb, making sleep harder, not easier. Connection, safety, and emotional comfort are key. The point isn't performance. It's presence. A comfortable, relaxed, emotionally connected encounter—whether sexual or simply affectionate—is one of nature's oldest and best sleep aids.

Final Thoughts (And a Little Homework)

So, if you're looking for a natural way to fall asleep tonight, you might want to skip the sleeping pills and consider another time-tested option. No side effects. No prescription required.

Go ahead and try this tonight. Class dismissed. You're welcome!

Eating Your Way to Better Sleep—or the Midnight Snack That Ruined Everything

"You are what you eat. So if you eat cookies at midnight, don't be surprised if you dream about being chased by Oreos." — Rogue Librarian Wisdom

It starts the same way every time. You're standing in the kitchen, refrigerator door open, bathed in the soft, judgmental glow of the lightbulb. The clock reads some ungodly hour, and your stomach is whispering sweet nothings about how a bowl of cereal might be the only thing standing between you and sweet, uninterrupted sleep. You give in. Ten minutes later, you're back in bed, but instead of drifting off, you're wide awake, acutely aware that you've made a terrible mistake.

Food and sleep have been tangled up together for as long as humans have been collapsing into heaps of straw at the end of a long day. Science, in its ever-enthusiastic pursuit of making things complicated, has spent decades dissecting this relationship, throwing around words like "circadian rhythm," "serotonin synthesis," and "glycemic variability." The short version is this: what you eat, when you eat it, and how much of it you stuff into your face all play a significant role in how well you sleep.

But fear not. Unlike most sleep advice, which seems to require you to either become a monk or give up coffee, this chapter will guide you toward practical, actionable dietary changes that actually make sense. No gimmicks. No magical superfoods. Just real, evidence-based strategies to turn your body into the well-oiled, sleep-friendly machine it was meant to be.

How Food Affects Sleep: The Science

The relationship between food and sleep hinges on a few key biological processes, none of which require a PhD in biochemistry to understand. At the center of it all is melatonin, the hormone we talked about earlier, which is responsible for making you sleepy. Your body produces melatonin naturally, but it needs the right building blocks to do so. This is where serotonin (a neurotransmitter that makes you feel content and relaxed) comes in, and serotonin, in turn, is synthesized from tryptophan, an amino acid found in certain foods.

Meanwhile, blood sugar stability also plays a crucial role. A massive spike in blood sugar, courtesy of a late-night sugar binge, might give you a brief energy boost, but the inevitable crash that follows can leave your body scrambling to balance things out, leading to disrupted sleep. The gut-brain axis—yes, your intestines and your brain talk to each other—further complicates the picture. A healthy gut microbiome has been linked to better sleep, while an imbalance can contribute to insomnia.

So, what does this mean for your plate? It means that the key to good sleep starts long before you even think about climbing into bed.

Key Nutrients for Sleep: The Dream Team

If you're looking to fine-tune your diet for better sleep, a few specific nutrients deserve your attention.

Magnesium: Think of magnesium as nature's muscle relaxant. It helps calm the nervous system, reduces stress, and has been shown to improve sleep quality. Leafy greens, nuts, seeds, and dark chocolate are good sources (and yes, this is a scientifically valid reason to eat the little chocolate square that the room steward on a cruise puts on your pillow before bed!).

Tryptophan: The amino acid that makes people blame Thanksgiving turkey for their post-meal comas. Tryptophan is a precursor to serotonin and melatonin, which means eating foods rich in it—like poultry, dairy, nuts, and seeds—can help set the stage for better sleep.

Omega-3s: Found in fatty fish, walnuts, and flaxseeds, omega-3 fatty acids reduce inflammation and support healthy brain function, which in turn promotes deeper, more restorative sleep.

B Vitamins: These little guys help regulate melatonin production. B6, found in bananas and poultry, is particularly important for converting tryptophan into serotonin.

The MIND Diet and Why It Works

There's a lot of dietary nonsense out there, but the MIND diet (a combination of the Mediterranean and DASH diets) actually holds up under scrutiny. Research suggests that following this diet improves overall sleep quality and even helps prevent cognitive decline.

The MIND diet focuses on brain-healthy foods like leafy greens, berries, nuts, whole grains, olive oil, and fatty fish, while cutting back on processed junk, butter, and too much red meat. Its emphasis on anti-inflammatory and antioxidant-rich foods supports the gut-brain axis and helps regulate sleep-related hormones.

Translation? Eating more spinach and salmon and fewer cheeseburgers and donuts could be the difference between deep, restorative sleep and another night of staring at the ceiling, questioning all your life choices.

The Worst Foods for Sleep: The Usual Suspects

You probably already suspect that a triple espresso at 9 p.m. isn't a recipe for sweet dreams, but some of the biggest sleep disruptors aren't quite as obvious.

High-Sugar Foods: That innocent-looking bowl of ice cream might be the reason you're waking up at 3 a.m. Sugar sends blood glucose levels soaring, followed by a sharp crash that signals your body to release cortisol, the stress hormone.

Fried and Fatty Foods: Late-night pizza might feel like a spiritual experience at the moment, but digesting high-fat meals requires a lot of energy, which can interfere with sleep quality.

Spicy Foods: Heartburn and restless sleep go hand in hand. If you enjoy spicy meals, consider having them earlier in the day.

Excessive Protein: Your body loves protein, but a huge steak right before bed makes digestion harder, which can interfere with sleep cycles. Balance is key.

Timing Matters: When You Eat is Just as Important as What You Eat

The timing of meals has a bigger impact on sleep than most people realize. Eating too close to bedtime —especially heavy or high-carb meals—can keep the digestive system working overtime when it should be slowing down.

On the other hand, going to bed too hungry can also backfire. Low blood sugar can trigger the release of cortisol, which keeps you awake. The sweet spot? Eating your last substantial meal 3-4 hours before bed and, if necessary, a light, sleep-friendly snack about 30 minutes before sleep.

Hydration, Caffeine, and Alcohol: The Sleep Wrecking Crew

Caffeine: If you're sensitive to caffeine, it's best to cut it off at least six hours before bed. That means no late-afternoon coffee or sneaky energy drinks.

Alcohol: The great deceiver. While alcohol might help you fall asleep faster, it significantly disrupts REM sleep, leading to grogginess the next day. If you drink, do so earlier in the evening and in moderation.

Hydration: Being dehydrated can cause nighttime leg cramps and general discomfort, but overdoing it on fluids before bed guarantees midnight bathroom trips. The fix? Hydrate well throughout the day but ease up a couple of hours before bedtime.

Practical Steps to Optimize Your Diet for Sleep

The way you eat throughout the day inevitably shapes the way you sleep at night. By now, it's clear that nutrition plays a direct role in everything from melatonin production to blood sugar stability, and even the gut-brain connection. But understanding the science is one thing—putting it into practice is another. The good news is that small, intentional shifts in your diet can make a real difference in how well you sleep.

Making changes to your diet doesn't have to be overwhelming. The first step is to prioritize foods that you like that naturally support sleep. Magnesium-rich leafy greens and nuts help relax muscles and calm the nervous system, while omega-3s from fatty fish reduce inflammation and improve sleep quality. Tryptophan, found in poultry, dairy, and seeds, provides the raw material your body needs to produce serotonin and melatonin, making it easier to fall asleep and stay asleep.

At the same time, cutting back on processed sugars and heavy, high-fat meals—especially in the evening —helps prevent the blood sugar spikes and digestive strain that often lead to restless nights. Timing matters just as much as content. Eating too late forces your body to stay in digestion mode when it should be winding down, while going to bed too hungry can trigger a stress response that keeps you awake. A balanced dinner, finished at least three hours before bedtime, gives your body the best chance at uninterrupted rest.

Caffeine and alcohol deserve special attention. While caffeine's stimulatory effects are obvious, its long half-life means that even an afternoon cup of coffee can interfere with sleep. Cutting it off by mid-afternoon is often enough to prevent unwanted wakefulness. Alcohol, on the other hand, masquerades as a sleep aid but ultimately disrupts REM sleep, leaving you groggy and unrefreshed in the morning.

For those times when a late-night craving strikes, the right kind of snack can actually help rather than hurt. A small handful of nuts, a serving of yogurt, or a bowl of oatmeal provides a steady source of nutrients that support sleep without causing disruptions. Making these simple dietary shifts isn't about perfection—it's about creating habits that set you up for better, more restorative sleep night after night.

Final Thoughts: You Are What You Eat (And How You Sleep)

Food is fuel, but it's also information. Every bite you take sends signals to your body, influencing not just how you feel during the day but how well you sleep at night. Small, consistent changes to your diet can transform your sleep quality, giving you the energy and clarity to tackle each day like the well-rested, unstoppable force you were meant to be.

If you're currently surviving on a diet of gas station snacks and takeout, don't panic. Progress, not perfection, is the goal. Make one change today, then another next week. Your future, well-rested self will thank you.

In the next chapter, we're tackling the physical side of sleep—your environment. Think of it like setting the stage for a great performance. Your body is the lead actor, but if the lighting's wrong, the background noise is chaos, and the set design screams "laundry pile," even the best performance is going to flop.

The truth is, your sleep space can either work with you or against you. If your bedroom feels like a Vegas casino, a polar expedition, or a multi-purpose storage room with a mattress in the middle, your brain's going to stay confused—and wide awake.

Ready to turn your room into an actual sleep-friendly space? Good. Let's give your environment the makeover it's been quietly begging for.

Your Bedroom Called...

"Nothing says 'restful oasis' like the glow of three screens and a pile of Amazon boxes."—Rogue Librarian Wisdom

You've started strong—moved your body and ate a sleep inducing turkey dinner. But if your sleep environment is working against you, all that effort can only take you so far. The truth is, your bedroom matters—a lot. If the space you're sleeping in feels more like a storage closet, a sauna, or a late-night entertainment center, your brain's going to have a hard time getting the memo that it's time to rest. To fall asleep easily and stay asleep, you need more than good habits—you need a space designed to support deep, uninterrupted sleep. Let's get that part right.

Here's the thing—sleep isn't just about what's happening in your brain. Your body is scanning the room like an overcaffeinated security guard, deciding if conditions are suitable for rest. Too much light? Too much noise? A mattress that feels suspiciously like an old canoe? Congratulations, you've just sabotaged your own sleep.

This chapter is about fixing all the things you don't realize are messing with your rest. Because the truth is, if your bedroom isn't designed for sleep, all the relaxation techniques in the world won't help. Let's turn your sleep space into a place where actual sleep happens—not just frustration, tossing, and dramatic sighing.

Most people assume that if they're tired enough, they'll fall asleep no matter what. They believe that the bedroom environment doesn't play a major role in sleep quality. They focus on what they do before bed but ignore the setting they're sleeping in. Then, when sleep remains elusive, they blame themselves, assuming something is wrong with their body or their mind.

A more effective approach is to recognize that the bedroom itself plays a significant role in sleep quality. The brain is highly sensitive to environmental cues, and even small disruptions—light, sound, temperature, discomfort—can keep it in a state of alertness. Fixing these issues creates an environment where sleep happens naturally rather than becoming a battle each night.

Optimizing Light for Better Sleep

The body's internal clock is directly influenced by light. Exposure to natural light in the morning helps regulate sleep-wake cycles, but just as importantly, reducing artificial light in the evening signals to the brain that it's time to wind down. Many people unknowingly sabotage their sleep by keeping their bedroom too bright at night. Even small sources of light—like alarm clocks, streetlights shining through the window, or the glow from a television—can disrupt melatonin production and make it harder to fall asleep.

Creating a truly dark sleep environment makes a noticeable difference. Blackout curtains block outside light, and removing or covering small light sources in the bedroom eliminates unnecessary disruptions. A bedside lamp with warm, dim lighting instead of overhead bright lights in the evening helps signal to the brain that it's time to prepare for rest. For those who need some light, using red-toned bulbs instead of blue or white light reduces melatonin suppression and keeps the brain in a relaxed state.

You should also know that, while we're on the topic of light, your smartphone has other plans—namely, bombarding your eyes with blue light that screams, "Stay awake!" Blue light, especially in the evening, can trick your brain into thinking it's still daytime, suppressing melatonin production and throwing your circadian rhythm out of whack.

But before you panic and banish all screens after sunset, it's worth noting that the brightness and duration of exposure play significant roles. According to Stuart Peirson, a professor of circadian neuroscience at Oxford University, while blue light does influence sleep, other wavelengths do too, and the overall brightness and exposure time are more critical factors.

So, instead of investing in blue light blocking glasses that may or may not work, consider reducing screen time before bed and lowering your device's brightness. After all, your social media feed will still be there in the morning, but your sleep won't wait.

Controlling Sound for Undisturbed Rest

Alright, so you've dimmed the lights, banished the blue glow of your phone, and set your bedroom up for peak sleep mode. But if your nighttime soundtrack consists of car alarms, your neighbor's late-night TV binge, or your partner sawing logs at a decibel level that should require a permit, we have another problem.

Even if you think you've "tuned out" the noise, your brain is still listening—like a paranoid security guard who refuses to clock out. Sudden or inconsistent sounds can yank you out of deep sleep, even if you don't fully wake up. And that means lower-quality rest and more groggy mornings.

So, what's the fix? Controlled sound. White noise machines, fans, or nature soundtracks create a steady hum that drowns out unpredictable noises. It's like an audio security blanket for your brain—keeping things consistent so it doesn't feel the need to jolt awake at every little disturbance. If you prefer pure silence, earplugs are your best friend (and possibly your marriage saver).

And then there's the stealth noise culprit—your beloved pet. Sure, they're adorable, but a dog shifting every ten minutes or a cat launching themselves off your dresser at 3 AM can add more disruptions than you realize. If your sleep feels restless but you can't figure out why, take a hard look at the furry suspect snoring beside you. No judgment if you keep them in the bed—just know they might be the reason you're not getting that deep, dream-filled slumber.

The goal here is simple: eliminate unpredictable noise. Because if you're waking up tired every morning, your sleep environment might be staging a sabotage mission—one beep, snore, or purring cat at a time.

The Great Sleep Temperature Debate: You vs. Your Blanket

Let's talk about one of the sneakiest sleep saboteurs out there—temperature. Most people don't realize that their bedroom is basically a slow cooker, trapping them in a night of sweaty, restless misery. The body naturally cools down to signal that it's time to sleep, but if your room feels like a summer afternoon in Florida, your brain is going to have some objections.

The ideal sleep temperature? Somewhere between 60-67°F (15-19°C)—cool enough to keep your body in its natural sleep zone, but not so cold that you shiver yourself awake.. Think *crisp fall morning*, not *meat locker*.

One common mistake is going full burrito mode with heavy blankets, only to wake up at 2 AM feeling like a microwaved Hot Pocket. Instead, opt for breathable bedding—moisture-wicking sheets, a lighter blanket, or even a cooling mattress topper. The goal is temperature regulation, not a nightly battle between being too hot under the covers and too cold when you stick one foot out.

Moral of the story? Your bedroom should feel cool, not tropical.

Choosing the Right Mattress and Pillow

A bad mattress or pillow doesn't just lead to discomfort—it actively prevents deep sleep. Many people assume that tossing and turning is just a normal part of sleep, but it's often a sign that their body is trying to compensate for an unsupportive sleep surface.

Over time, this leads to back pain, stiffness, and fragmented sleep cycles. A mattress that is too soft can cause the body to sink in too much, leading to misalignment, while one that is too firm can create pressure points.

The right mattress supports the spine while allowing for enough cushioning to reduce discomfort. Similarly, the right pillow depends on sleep position. Side sleepers need thicker pillows for neck support, while back sleepers benefit from thinner pillows that keep the head aligned with the spine.

People who wake up with pain or stiffness should assess whether their mattress and pillow might be contributing to their sleep issues. Even small changes, like adding a mattress topper or adjusting pillow height, can make a noticeable difference.

Common Mistakes That Sabotage the Sleep Environment

One of the most frequent mistakes people make is assuming that if they're tired enough, they'll sleep anywhere. While exhaustion can override some discomfort, poor sleep environments lead to more

fragmented sleep and more wake-ups throughout the night. Another mistake is leaving electronics in the bedroom. Even if a TV is turned off, the association between the bedroom and entertainment rather than rest makes it harder to mentally unwind.

Some people also make the mistake of keeping the bedroom cluttered. A messy room creates a subconscious sense of chaos, making it harder for the brain to fully relax. Keeping the bedroom simple, organized, and dedicated solely to sleep reinforces the connection between the environment and rest.

A Simple Change to Try Tonight

Tonight, before bed, take five minutes to assess the bedroom. Turn off all lights and check for any sources of artificial brightness. Listen for noises that might be disrupting sleep, whether it's an air conditioner that cycles too loudly or distant street noise. Adjust the temperature to the cooler side and make sure the bedding allows for comfort without overheating. Small adjustments can lead to immediate improvements in sleep quality.

Reinforcing a Sleep-Friendly Space

Creating an optimal sleep environment isn't about luxury—it's about functionality. Light, sound, temperature, and comfort all send powerful signals to your body that it's time to sleep.

When you get these basics right, your bedroom stops being another source of stress and starts becoming what it was always meant to be: a place of real rest. Of course, even the perfect sleep cave can't shut down a brain that's still buzzing like a neon sign at midnight.

If you've ever found yourself physically exhausted but mentally wired—spinning through to-do lists, arguments, random grocery items, and the embarrassing thing you said in third grade—you're not alone.

That's where we're headed next: how to break the "Tired But Wired" cycle and finally give your brain the green light to sleep

Breaking The "Tired But Wired" Cycle

"Sometimes the most productive thing you can do is take a nap and stop trying to control the universe."
— Anonymous

There's a moment every insomniac dreads. It's that second wind that kicks in just as they were supposed to be getting sleepy. The day has been spent feeling sluggish, chugging coffee, and fantasizing about sleep, yet the moment the head hits the pillow, the body and brain snap to full attention.

Suddenly, sleep isn't an option. Thoughts fire in every direction, and the energy that was so desperately missing all day has arrived at precisely the wrong time. This is the "tired but wired" cycle, and it's one of the biggest reasons people struggle with insomnia.

The most common reaction? Trying to force sleep. People lie in bed, willing themselves into unconsciousness, convinced that if they just stay still long enough, sleep will happen.

It doesn't work. Sleep isn't something you can muscle your way into—it's something your body has to naturally ease into. The harder you fight, the more awake you become. Frustration builds, bedtime feels stressful, and the cycle deepens.

Another misfire is pushing through exhaustion all day, believing that the body will eventually "crash" at night. This often leads to over-caffeination, skipped breaks, and nonstop stimulation—basically sending your brain the message to stay on high alert.

You've already heard me say it once (or maybe a dozen times), but it's worth repeating: sleep is a full-day process.

The way you move, eat, think, and light yourself throughout the day either sets you up for a smooth landing at night—or a crash-and-burn.

Instead of rehashing every detail about circadian rhythms, daylight exposure, and screens (been there, done that, got the T-shirt), let's zoom in on why this matters so much when you're stuck in the "tired but wired" loop—and how to actually break free.

Resetting the Internal Clock

By now, you know that your internal clock runs on light. Morning light resets it; nighttime light scrambles it.

If you've been following along, you already know the drill: sunlight early, dim light late, screens down before bed.

What's different here is **why** it's so important for the "wired at night" feeling: your brain gets completely confused if it misses the daytime signals.

Starting tomorrow, step outside within an hour of waking up—rain or shine—and get some real light.

You're not just checking a box. You're giving your brain the "wake up now" cue it desperately needs, which makes the "sleep later" cue possible.

Increasing Natural Sleep Pressure

Sleep pressure is the buildup of tiredness throughout the day. It's what makes sleep feel irresistible at night. When sleep pressure is too low, the body doesn't feel tired enough to fall asleep easily. The problem is that many modern habits interfere with this natural process. Napping for too long, staying sedentary, and drinking too much caffeine late in the day all reduce sleep pressure, leading to the dreaded "wide awake at bedtime" feeling.

In a previous chapter, we discussed how physical activity plays a major role in building sleep pressure. People who move their bodies regularly throughout the day fall asleep faster and experience deeper, more restorative sleep. Exercise, particularly in the morning or early afternoon, increases sleep drive, making nighttime rest more natural. Even a simple 20-minute walk outside can make a noticeable difference in how the body transitions to sleep.

Caffeine also plays a significant role. While a morning coffee is fine, caffeine lingers in the system for hours. Many people underestimate its impact and drink coffee, tea, or energy drinks in the afternoon, unaware that caffeine remains in the bloodstream for up to ten hours. Cutting off caffeine intake by early afternoon prevents it from interfering with the body's natural wind-down process.

Breaking the Cycle of Overstimulation

This one's a biggie. Most people spend their evenings absorbing stress and stimulation like a sponge—intense shows, rapid scrolling, heated debates about whose turn it is to take out the trash.

Here's the brutal truth: your brain can't slam the brakes from "full speed ahead" to "peaceful slumber" in five minutes. You need a wind-down runway. Same activities, same order, every night.

Dim the lights. Pick up a book. Stretch a little. Listen to something calming. You're basically training your brain to recognize, "Oh hey, sleep's coming," instead of "Let's solve world peace right now!"

Common Mistakes That Keep People Stuck

One of the biggest mistakes people make is trying to "fix" sleep by sleeping in longer. While it seems logical to catch up on lost sleep, inconsistent wake-up times throw off the body's internal clock and make it harder to feel naturally sleepy the next night. A consistent wake-up time, even on weekends, reinforces the body's natural rhythm and makes it easier to fall asleep at the right time.

Another mistake is relying on naps to make up for poor nighttime sleep. While short naps can be beneficial, long naps—especially in the late afternoon—reduce the body's sleep pressure, making it harder to fall asleep at night. Keeping naps under

30 minutes and limiting them to earlier in the day helps maintain a healthy sleep cycle.

Some people also make the mistake of trying to tire themselves out by staying up as late as possible. This backfires because it disrupts the body's natural rhythm and increases stress levels. A better approach is to maintain a regular bedtime and focus on habits that naturally increase sleep pressure throughout the day.

A Simple Exercise to Start Resetting Sleep

Tomorrow morning, get outside early. Pair it with something you like—walking, listening to a podcast, or just enjoy a cup of coffee outside—and make it enjoyable, not a chore.

You're not just chasing light; you're teaching your body when to feel awake—and when not to.

Reinforcing the New Sleep Cycle

Breaking the "tired but wired" cycle isn't about brute force. It's about creating the right conditions so your body can follow its natural rhythms—without you wrestling it every night.

Reset your clock. Build your sleep pressure. Ease off the stimulation. Done consistently, sleep starts to happen on its own, the way it's supposed to.

So, your body's tired but your brain missed the memo and is still hosting a late-night brainstorming session. Classic.

In the next chapter, we're going straight to the source of that "tired but wired" feeling—your overactive, opinionated, won't-stop-talking brain.

We'll unpack why it won't settle down and walk through a surprisingly simple formula to help you shut off the mental noise and finally ease into sleep.

Ready to learn how to outsmart your own mind? Turn the page. Your brain won't know what hit it.

The "Mind Off" Formula – Stopping Racing Thoughts At Night

"Dear Brain, if you don't shut up, we're both going to suffer tomorrow." — Rogue Librarian Wisdom

Here's the frustrating truth about sleep: if sleep was an animal, it would be a cat. You can beg, plead, count sheep, or even threaten, but sleep shows up when it wants to, not when you call it. The trick isn't to chase it but to set the right conditions so it comes padding into the room willingly.

In the last chapter, we covered how sleep isn't just something that magically happens at bedtime—it's the grand finale of a whole day's worth of preparation. Resetting your body's internal clock, building up natural sleep pressure, and avoiding overstimulation all play a part in making sleep easier.

But what if you do everything right and your body is exhausted, yet your brain refuses to get the memo? The moment your head hits the pillow, your brain suddenly decides it's the perfect time to relive embarrassing moments from middle school or map out an elaborate plan for reorganizing the garage.

The thoughts begin small. Maybe a stray worry about something that didn't get finished during the day. Then it expands. An old memory. A cringeworthy moment from five years ago. The grocery list. A sudden urge to solve a problem that could easily wait until morning. Thoughts spiral and multiply, and before long, what should have been a restful transition into sleep has turned into a full-blown mental marathon.

Many people attempt to fight these thoughts by trying to forcibly push them away. This never works. The more someone tells their brain to be quiet, the louder it becomes. Others attempt to distract themselves with screens, watching TV, scrolling their phone, or listening to a podcast in the hopes that background noise will override their own mind. While this can sometimes work temporarily, it creates a dependency that ultimately makes falling asleep without these crutches even harder.

So what's the solution? You need a way to shut down your brain as effectively as your body. The problem is not that the mind is active; the problem is that it has been conditioned to be active at the wrong time. Changing this requires breaking the habit of mentally rehearsing worries in bed and giving the brain an alternative, structured way to unwind.

Clearing Mental Clutter Before Bed

The brain does not like unfinished business. If the mind is racing at night, it is often because there are unresolved thoughts that haven't been processed properly. One of the simplest ways to address this is to create a designated time before bed to offload thoughts onto paper.

A simple exercise that has been proven to reduce sleep latency is writing down everything that is on the mind. This is not the same as keeping a traditional journal or writing in long, structured sentences. It's a raw brain dump. Bullet points, single words, scattered thoughts—everything that is floating around in the head should go onto paper. The goal is not to organize these thoughts or even come up with solutions. The goal is simply to take them out of the brain and put them somewhere else.

People who do this often find that their minds quiet down significantly when they get into bed. Instead of worrying about forgetting something important, they know that anything worth remembering has already been written down. The brain feels safer letting go.

Training the Brain to Recognize Sleep Signals

Sleep is a habit. Just like people can train themselves to crave coffee in the morning or feel hungry at certain times of the day, they can also train their brains to associate specific signals with sleep. Right now, many people have trained their brains to associate bedtime with stress. The moment they lie down, their brain interprets it as a cue to start running through every unfinished thought. This is a learned response, and just like any habit, it can be rewired.

One of the most effective ways to do this is by creating a structured pre-bedtime routine. This doesn't have to be elaborate. It simply needs to be a repeatable sequence of calming activities that the brain begins to associate with sleep. Stretching, reading, dimming the lights, deep breathing—when done consistently in the same order every night, these activities send a strong signal that sleep is coming. Over time, the brain will start responding by automatically shifting into a more relaxed state.

I'd also like to point out that this focus on routine is one of the best ways to help children prepare for bedtime as well. Make the routine fun for them and it will be an enjoyable time rather than a battle. One of my sons starts his daughter's night time routine with a race up the stairs to her bedroom. He always lets her win—but just barely.

Redirecting Thoughts with Guided Relaxation

For those who struggle with particularly stubborn racing thoughts, adding a mental relaxation technique can help redirect the brain's activity. One of the most effective methods is progressive muscle relaxation. It is part of the Military Method, which we will cover in detail in the next chapter. This technique involves systematically tensing and then relaxing different muscle groups, starting from the toes and working up to the head. This not only helps release physical tension but also gives the brain a structured focus, preventing it from drifting into anxious thought patterns.

Another effective strategy is visualization. Instead of allowing the mind to wander aimlessly, directing it toward a calming mental image—like a slow-moving river, a peaceful forest, or even a simple counting exercise—can guide it toward a state of relaxation. The key is consistency. Just as the mind has been trained to race at night, it can be trained to slow down when given the right cues.

One other method I turn to—especially when my brain decides it's going to stage a mental protest at 11:47 p.m.—is Scripture. Specifically, *Philippians 4:6–7*, which has gotten me through more than a few sleepless nights.

> *"Do not be anxious about anything, but in every situation, by prayer and petition, with thanksgiving, present your requests to God. And the peace of God, which transcends all understanding, will guard your hearts and your minds in Christ Jesus."*
>
> *New International Version (NIV)*

As a Christian, I often turn to the Bible when life gets complicated. This particular verse has become my go-to when my thoughts start doing cartwheels and won't stop. It's a reminder that I don't have to carry all the weight on my own shoulders. I can hand those anxious thoughts over to God—every last one of them—and trust Him to handle what I can't.

And here's the part that gets me every time: the promise. Not just peace—but *peace that transcends all understanding.* Not logical, not explainable, not tied to circumstances. Just peace. The kind that wraps around your racing mind and says, *"I've got this. You can rest now."*

Even if you're not particularly religious, there's something powerful about releasing your worries—especially through prayer. For me, knowing that I'm handing them over to a God who loves me and is actually capable of doing something about them—that's the most reassuring sleep strategy I've ever found. And hey—who wouldn't want an all-powerful, all-loving God standing guard over their thoughts while they sleep? Seems like a pretty solid upgrade from white noise.

Common Pitfalls and How to Avoid Them

One of the most common mistakes people make when trying to quiet their minds is treating relaxation techniques as another task to complete. If an approach doesn't work immediately, frustration sets in, making relaxation even more difficult. The key is to approach these techniques with patience and consistency. The goal is not instant success but gradual improvement over time.

Another mistake is relying too heavily on distractions. Using white noise or calming sounds can be helpful, but they should not become a requirement for sleep. The ultimate goal is to be able to fall asleep naturally, without needing an external crutch.

Finally, many people assume that if they still have racing thoughts after implementing these strategies, they are doing something wrong. This is not the case. The brain is designed to think. The goal is not to eliminate thoughts altogether but to create a more structured, calming approach to how those thoughts are managed at night.

A Simple Practice to Try Tonight

Before bed, try the "Three-Box Mental Dump." Grab a notebook (or your phone, if you promise not to start scrolling) and divide your thoughts into three mental "boxes": *Stuff I Need to Deal With, Stuff I Can't Control,* and *Random Nonsense That Won't Shut Up.*

Dump every lingering thought into the right category. That email you forgot to send? It goes in *Need to Deal With.* Worrying about the stock market or the weather next week? Straight into *Can't*

Control. That weird, looping memory of an awkward conversation from five years ago? Yep, that belongs in *Random Nonsense*.

Once you've sorted it all out, close the notebook and tell yourself, *"That's handled. Brain, your shift is over."* Then, when you get into bed and a stray thought tries to sneak back in, remind yourself that it's already been filed away. Pair this with slow breathing or a body scan, and let your mind clock out for the night.

Use a simple mantra like "not now, time to rest" whenever your mind starts revving back up. The goal isn't to erase all thoughts but to create a system that signals your brain that it's officially clock-out time.

Over time, this practice helps train your brain to stop its nighttime overthinking habit—because let's be honest, 2 AM is never the time for brilliant problem-solving anyway.

Stopping racing thoughts is not about suppressing them; it is about giving the brain a different process to follow. By clearing mental clutter before bed, creating a structured wind-down routine, and using guided relaxation techniques, it becomes easier to break free from the cycle of nighttime overthinking.

The Next Step Toward Better Sleep

Let's be honest—calming the mind at night is a skill most of us never learned. We were taught how to parallel park, memorize the periodic table, and pretend to enjoy kale... but no one pulled us aside and said, *"Here's what to do when your brain refuses to shut up at bedtime."*

Back at the beginning of the book, in *Sleep Triage,* I said there were two chapters I send people to when they're tired, desperate, and just want something that *works*. You're about to read one of them. It's the sleep method that's helped soldiers fall asleep in chaos, and now it's about to become your secret weapon.

If you're ready for a step-by-step method to fall asleep faster and train your body to shut down on cue, this is it.

Turn the page. Let's get to the good stuff.

The Military Method: Falling Asleep Like a Soldier

Discipline is choosing between what you want now and what you want most. Like, sleep." — Abraham Lincoln (adapted)

Okay, two things before we get started.

First, have you created the best environment possible for the space you sleep in? Is it dark, cool and quiet?

Second, Is your body tired? Maybe you went for a walk, did some squats while waiting for your coffee to brew, or chased your dog around the yard like a lunatic. Good. Your body needs to earn its rest.

But here's the thing—just because you're physically tired doesn't mean your brain got the memo.

That's where this next trick comes in. It's a method so effective, so battle-tested, that it was literally developed for soldiers and pilots.

If it works for them, it can work for you, even if your biggest sleep threat is an overactive mind and a particularly enthusiastic group chat.

The Backstory: How the Military Cracked the Sleep Code

Imagine your day job is in the cockpit of a fighter jet, or on the battlefield where people are actively trying to kill you. High stress, running on barely any sleep, adrenaline pumping, and knowing that one wrong move could get you (and a lot of other people) into serious trouble. Not exactly the ideal conditions for drifting off into peaceful slumber, right?

The U.S. military realized that sleep deprivation was a major problem—one that led to poor decisions, slowed reflexes, and mistakes they couldn't afford. So, they developed a system to help military personnel fall asleep fast, no matter where they were. The result? The Military Method, a simple routine designed to knock you out in two minutes or less. That's right—two minutes. The time it takes to microwave a Hot Pocket.

Now, I know what you're thinking. *Yeah, right. If this worked, I wouldn't be reading a book about sleep.* I get it. But stay with me.

How the Military Method Works (Step-by-Step Guide)

Here's the process, straight from the people who perfected the fine art of sleeping under extreme conditions:

1. Relax your face – Every part of it. That means unclenching your jaw, letting your tongue drop from the roof of your mouth, and releasing the tension you didn't even know you were holding in your forehead. Yes, that permanent squint you've developed from staring at screens counts.

2. Drop your shoulders – You are not trying to wear them as earrings. Let them sink down and melt into whatever surface you're lying on. Feel them go heavy.

3. Relax your arms – Start at the hands. Let them go limp. Then the forearms. Then the upper arms. Let them flop like overcooked spaghetti.

4. Exhale and relax your chest – Take a deep breath in. Then let it out slowly, like you're dramatically sighing at a long customer service hold time. Feel your chest sink and let your breathing slow naturally.

5. Relax your legs – Same deal as the arms. Start at the thighs and work your way down to your feet, letting each muscle group go slack. Your legs should feel like someone swapped them out for bags of wet sand.

6. Clear your mind – This is the hardest part, but it's key. Go to your happy place mentally. Picture something peaceful, like floating on a calm lake or lying in a meadow. Mine is sitting on a dune at Lake Michigan and looking out at the lake. If your brain won't cooperate and insists on thinking about that embarrassing thing you said in 2004, try repeating a simple phrase. You can make up your own or try "I am *going to sleep now"* to yourself.

That's it. Stick with it, and in about two minutes, your body will take over and do what it's supposed to and go to sleep.

Why This Method Works

The Military Method isn't magic—it's science. It forces your body into a state of progressive relaxation, short-circuiting the stress response that keeps you awake. It also gives your brain something to focus on other than, say, your growing to-do list or whether or not you locked the front door (you did).

And here's the best part: It works anywhere. On a plane, on a couch, in the middle of a noisy apartment building where your neighbor insists on vacuuming at midnight. It doesn't require equipment, supplements, or complete silence—just a little practice.

Here's a fun little story. My wife, Kate, was proofreading this book out loud to me as we drove— once again—to yet another one of our grandkids' soccer games.

Somewhere between merging onto the freeway and searching for the right field on Google Maps, she reached this chapter. She started reading through the list of relaxation steps, nice and steady, just like she had been with the rest of the book. But then something changed. Midway through the list… she yawned. And then yawned again. And again. Pretty soon, she could barely get through a sentence without another yawn sneaking in.

Now, was it just coincidence? Or is this chapter actually *that* relaxing?

You be the judge. (But maybe don't read it while driving.)

Try This Tonight: Your Two-Minute Sleep Challenge

Let's put this thing to the test. Tonight, when you lie down, run through the steps. Give yourself two full minutes to let it work. If you're still awake after that, try it again.

The key is consistency. Just like training for anything else, the more you do it, the better your body gets at responding. Soldiers don't master this on their first try—but once they do, they can sleep anywhere, anytime, even in the middle of chaos.

And let's be honest, your bedroom—no matter how bad your insomnia—is probably not as intense as a battlefield.

Closing Thought: Sleep Is a Skill, Not Just Luck

The Military Method proves something important: sleep isn't just some mysterious force you either have or don't. It's a skill. One you can train for, practice, and improve. If soldiers can learn to fall asleep in war zones, you can learn to do it in the comfort of your own bed.

Warning: This method takes practice—but fast results are common. So go practice your two-minute knockout routine. You've got this.

The 5-Step Nighttime Routine That Signals "Sleep Mode"

"Routine is not a cage; it's a key to freedom. Especially freedom from staring at your ceiling at 3 a.m." — Rogue Librarian Wisdom

We've covered a lot in this book—probably more than you ever expected to know about sleep. Welcome to my world. Now, it's time to pull it all together. This chapter is your grand finale, the part where we take everything you've learned and turn it into a personalized sleep routine that actually works in real life for you. Not just "ideas," but a repeatable, real-world, fits-your-life kind of plan.

Let's get something straight right up front: sleep doesn't just happen because you're tired. Exhaustion might make you want to sleep, but it doesn't guarantee it. Sleep needs signals. It needs an intentional transition. If your entire day is go-go-go and then you expect your body to flip a switch the second your head hits the pillow—well, you already know how that story ends– you, staring at the ceiling, wondering what went wrong.

This is where your night time routine comes in. Not some strange bedtime ritual with candles and chanting (unless you're into that), but a real pattern your brain can count on. When your evenings are predictable, your body knows what to do. The key is to stop sending mixed messages—like scrolling on your phone in bed and expecting your brain to interpret that as "relaxation."

So what does this magical, non-magical routine actually look like?

First, you need to cut the mental chaos. That means shutting down the stimulation machine—work, screens, stressful conversations, and anything that revs you up. Give your brain at least an hour to understand that the day is winding down. If you're still answering emails or watching dramatic plot twists at 9:59 p.m., don't be surprised if your body isn't ready for lights out at 10.

Second, lighting matters more than you think. Your brain responds to light like a sunflower—it stays alert when the lights are blazing. If your house is lit up like a department store after hours, melatonin production doesn't stand a chance. Switch to soft, warm light in the evening. It tells your body, without you saying a word, that bedtime is coming.

Third, your activities need to change gears. If your wind-down routine currently involves "just checking one more thing" or watching a cooking show that makes you want to get up and bake banana bread at midnight, it's time for a swap. You want calming, repetitive activities—stretching, reading, quiet music, even just sitting in low light doing nothing in particular. The goal here isn't to do something productive. It's to send your nervous system the message: we're safe, we're slowing down, and no one's asking for anything right now.

Fourth, use sleep cues. These are the little rituals your body learns to associate with shutting down. Think of them like a sleep signal your brain can't ignore. A warm shower is an excellent one—because when your body cools down afterward, it mimics the natural temperature drop that precedes sleep. Pajamas, herbal tea, a consistent bedtime—these aren't just quaint ideas. They're pattern-builders. And your brain thrives on patterns.

Fifth, and this one's big—don't get in bed until you're truly sleepy. Not just tired from a long day, but genuinely ready to sleep. Heavy eyelids, slow thoughts, the sensation of your body asking for rest. That's the signal. If you get in bed too early, hoping sleep will come find you, you're more likely to reinforce the habit of lying awake. Instead, stay up a little longer in your wind-down zone until that unmistakable sleepy feeling shows up. Then—and only then—get into bed.

That's it. The five steps: shut down stimulation, lower the lights, change gears, use sleep cues, and wait for real sleepiness. Done consistently, this routine becomes a powerful system your brain and body will start to follow almost automatically. You're not forcing sleep—you're creating the conditions that make it happen naturally.

Now, one last thing before we wrap up. Knowing how to signal "sleep mode" is powerful. But knowledge without action? That's just another forgotten TED Talk.

This is where you take what you've learned—the good, the bad, and the surprisingly simple—and actually shape it into something that works for you.

I've created a bonus resource to help do exactly that. It's a simple guide called *The Sleep Routine*

Worksheet and you can use it to design a night time routine that fits your life, your schedule, and yes, even your late-night cravings for "just one more episode. You'll find it in the Bonus Sleep Toolkit, which can be accessed by scanning the code on the Bonus Page at the front of this book.

Picture this: waking up tomorrow rested—not because you got lucky, but because you *planned* for it. That's what this worksheet is for. It's free, it's fast, and it might just be the smartest thing you do today. Grab it now before life distracts you with another "urgent" notification.

And speaking of turning good ideas into real sleep... in the next chapter, I'm going to show you how I went from tossing and turning to sleeping like one of Hemingway's cats sprawled in the sun—deep, content, and almost obnoxiously peaceful. Spoiler alert: it didn't involve fancy gadgets, miracle supplements, or sleeping upside down like a bat.

Turn the page for a Librarian SuperHero sleep saga.

How I Sleep Like Hemingway's Cats in the Sunshine

"Cats have it figured out. Sleep when you're tired. Eat when you're hungry. Ignore everyone when you feel like it." — Anonymous

I'll admit it: writing this chapter makes me a little shy. Sharing personal stuff—especially about how I sleep—feels a bit like leaving the bathroom door wide open when guests are over. It's not exactly scandalous, but it's more exposure than I'm usually aiming for.

Still, I think it's worth it. Books like this tend to make you feel like you know the author a little, and many of you have told me that it feels more like we're sitting down for coffee than you're slogging through a textbook. I like that. I like making new friends.

So, in the spirit of friendship, I'm going to pull back the curtain on my own sleep journey. I hope it helps.

And if at any point it feels like I'm oversharing, I apologize in advance.

First off, it's important to say that while I offer a lot of strategies in this book, I don't use every single one myself. I don't have to. My goal was always to create a book that's like a really great diner menu: you pick what looks good to you and leave the liver and onions for someone else.

Here's what I've got cooking in my own sleep kitchen.

For starters, I track my sleep and activity. I used to wear a Fitbit, which I loved, until it died a tragic, untimely death. (RIP, little buddy.) In a rush before a big hiking trip, I grabbed a cheaper wrist device that did the basics: track steps, heart rate, sleep, and not fall apart in a week. It's not the Cadillac of trackers, but it does the job—and honestly, you don't need to mortgage the house for a fancy wristband to get good data.

There are a bunch of options out there, and maybe someday I'll write a guide about them, but for now just know you can find great ones at all kinds of price points. I'll drop a few Amazon links in the Sleep Resources for those who like to window shop.

I sleep in a cool, dark, quiet room. Think arctic fox den, minus the actual foxes. Kate and I sleep under a quilt even in the summer because, as it turns out, being a little chilly makes for excellent snoozing. No bright blinking lights, no electronic buzzing, no neighborhood dogs barking... just a peaceful environment that whispers, *sleep now, human.*

My bed is comfortable. I know that sounds obvious, but you'd be amazed how many people are trying to sleep on what feels like a medieval torture device. I have a pillow that keeps my head nicely aligned with my spine since I'm a back sleeper, and if you don't think that matters, just try waking up with a neck crick that makes you feel like you lost a bar fight.

I also use a CPAP for sleep apnea. It's not exactly a fashion statement, but it has made a huge difference. The steady, soft hum of the CPAP machine and the gentle flow of air into my nostrils have become part of my nightly "we're going to sleep now" ritual.

Even though having something strapped to your face isn't the most comfortable thing in the world, it's become a soothing part of my regular night time routine that signals to my body that we're done adulting for the day. I don't just barrel into bed after a Netflix binge and expect magic to happen. No, my body needs a wind-down. A gentle shifting of gears from *go-go-go* to *slow-slow-slow*.

Physical exercise is a huge part of my sleep success. My exercise varies. I ride the bike at the gym. I use the elliptical and the treadmill. I golf, and when I'm flying solo, I walk the course with a pushcart like a respectable throwback to the good old days. I hike the trail behind my house, and when I have the time, I disappear for 2-3 hours and cover 7+ miles.

Long-distance hiking is one of my interests and I try to accomplish a longer trail or section of one every year. I've walked across Michigan—from Lake Huron to Lake Michigan, and from the Ohio border up to the Mackinac Bridge, and beyond to Lake Superior. We usually hike 10-15 miles a day when we're on a longer trail. On those days, sleep comes easily.

When I write, I use a standing desk. (And occasionally sit down because let's be honest, even standing can get old after a while.) Staying active throughout the day means my body actually *wants* to rest at night, not rebel and throw a midnight party.

Food is another piece of the puzzle. I aim to eat nutritious meals and—this is the hard part—stop eating 2–3 hours before bed. I'm still working on that one. Some nights the cheese drawer calls my name like a siren on the rocks, but I do my best to resist.

Mentally, I use a technique that is a rogue version of the Military Method to fall asleep. Funny thing—I didn't even know about the Military Method until I started digging into research for this book. "Fall asleep in two minutes flat" caught my attention (because, come on, wouldn't you click on that too?) and down the rabbit hole I went. As it turns out, my own method wasn't too far off.

I used to picture myself lying on a swimming dock at a summer camp where I worked as a lifeguard. Sun on my face, the dock gently rocking, the lapping of the water against the sides... pure bliss. Any calm mental image will do. Earlier in the book, I mentioned another one I use sometimes: sitting on a dune by Lake Michigan, watching a storm flash lightning way out over the lake—the same dune where I proposed to Kate.

When rogue thoughts—anxieties, worries, stray ideas about whether I left the garage door open—try to invade, I pull out the big guns: Philippians 4:6–7.

I pray. I give my worries to God, trusting that He's better equipped to handle them than I am at 2 a.m.

And the results? They're good. Like, really good. I usually fall asleep in under five minutes—okay, maybe six or seven on the rare night when my brain insists on an encore performance—but it's not often I'm still awake after ten. My tracker backs this up. I regularly log between eight and ten hours of sleep a night, with two to four hours of deep sleep and around three to five hours of light sleep. I usually only wake up once, and sometimes not at all.

Now, I know what you're thinking: *That's nice, but where's the proof?* Well, since I like to practice what I preach (and because I knew you might be a little suspicious), I submit the following chart from my sleep app:

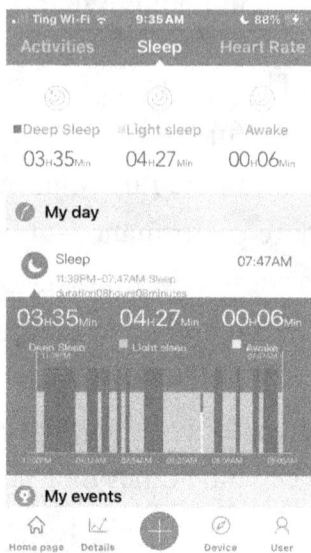

■Deep Sleep ▪Light sleep Awake
03ₕ35ₘᵢₙ 04ₕ27ₘᵢₙ 00ₕ06ₘᵢₙ

🕐 **My day**

🌙 Sleep   07:47AM
11:39PM~07:47AM Sleep
duration08hours08minutes

03ₕ35ₘᵢₙ 04ₕ27ₘᵢₙ 00ₕ06ₘᵢₙ

Deep Sleep   ▪Light sleep   ■Awake

💡 **My events**

🏠 Home page   📈 Details   ⊕   🧭 Device   👤 User

*Scientific evidence that adrenaline,
nachos, and questionable refereeing
decisions are no match for a good sleep
routine.*

And no, this wasn't on some boring Tuesday night.
This was the night of the NCAA Men's Basketball
Tournament Finals. If you're not a basketball fan,
just picture whatever would make your heart rate tap
dance right before bed. Florida won by 2 points—
right at the buzzer—and let's just say it wasn't
exactly a peaceful lead-up to lights out.

Even with all that excitement, the chart tells the real story: I fell asleep fast, clocked 3 hours and 35 minutes of deep sleep, 4 hours and 27 minutes of light sleep, and only spent six minutes awake (most of it probably trying to believe the game was actually over). I got up once in the middle of the night but went right back to sleep like a champ.

So yes, in the most humble, non-gloaty way possible... I told you I was a great sleeper. *Cue sheepish grin and a modest shrug. (Neener, Neener!)*

Before we move on, I need to hit pause for a moment. What comes next might be one of the most important parts of this entire book—for some of you, it might be *the* most important part.

Because if you've been reading along thinking, "Okay, I've tried the wind-down routines, I've dimmed the lights, I've sniffed the lavender, and I'm still waking up feeling like a half-charged phone from 2012," then this is for you.

It's easy to assume your sleep issues are just bad habits, too much stress, or maybe even a personal flaw (spoiler alert: they're not). But sometimes—and this is the part that matters—sometimes it's something medical. And if that's the case, no amount of warm baths or journaling is going to fix it.

So before we dig into more routines or clever tricks, I want to tell you a personal story. It's about the day I found out that my "normal" tiredness was anything but. And it all started with a meeting, a nap I didn't mean to take, and…

The Day My Boss Saved My Life (And Didn't Even Know It)

It happened on a Tuesday. Or maybe a Thursday. The kind of day where the clock moves like molasses and your coffee gives up trying to help around 10:17 a.m. We were in a staff meeting, and apparently, I was too.

What I remember is sitting there, nodding politely, doing my best to look interested while someone debated the urgent matter of creating a district wide formative assessment fidelity framework for calibration purposes (Are teachers really *formatively assessing*, or are they just *collecting data*? And how can we tell without a 12-question rubric?).

What my boss remembers is me nodding off—mid-sentence, mid-meeting, mid-life. Eyes closed, head tilted like a tranquilized bobblehead.

After the meeting, he pulled me aside. Not to reprimand me, bless him—but with genuine concern. He said, "Hey... I've noticed you seem exhausted all the time. You okay?" And then, after a pause that meant business:

"You might want to get checked out. This doesn't seem normal."

That moment stuck.

Because here's the thing: I *was* tired all the time. Bone-deep, dragging-a-cement-truck-uphill kind of tired. I thought I was just overworked, under-caffeinated, and maybe edging into the 'grumpy old man yells at clouds' stage of life. But something in his voice made me pause. And thank God it did.

Fast-forward a few weeks and a very glamorous overnight sleep study later (yes, I got to sleep in a room full of wires attached to every part of my body like some cyborg test subject from a low-budget sci-fi film), and the results were in.

Sleep apnea. A doozy of a case, too.

Apparently, I stopped breathing more often than a toddler who just learned the word 'why'. No wonder I felt like I'd been hit by a truck every morning. I wasn't getting rest—I was running nightly marathons in respiratory survival.

Now listen closely, friend: if there's even a flicker of suspicion in your gut that your exhaustion isn't normal—if you're sleeping all night and still waking up like a zombie with a coffee dependency—it's time to get checked.

I say that not as a doctor (obviously), but as someone who knows what it's like to think you're just "a tired person"... when in fact, your body is waving red flags and hoping you'll notice.

This chapter isn't the full story of my sleep apnea journey. That deserves its own book—and I'm writing that one too, for the brave souls who just got diagnosed and feel like they've been sentenced to a lifetime of sleeping with a leaf blower duct-taped to their face.

But this? This is the wake-up call I got. From a boss who cared enough to say something. From a sleep study that gave me answers. And from a machine I now sleep with every night that quite literally helps me breathe.

Moral of the story? Don't sleep on your symptoms. Get checked. See a sleep specialist. Don't wait for your boss to stage an intervention—or worse, for something serious to happen first.

Because the truth is, a good night's sleep starts with knowing what's *really* going on when your eyes are closed. And for some of us, the biggest sleep problem isn't the mattress, the lighting, or the caffeine. It's something deeper. Fixable, yes. But only if you know it's there.

So please—get checked.

Even if you don't fall asleep in meetings. (Though if you do, maybe don't sit directly across from your boss.)

So there you have it: my sleep life, laid bare. I hope this gives you a little hope and a lot of encouragement. Sleep problems aren't permanent, and while no two journeys are exactly the same, there's always a path forward. If I can get from bleary-eyed exhaustion to consistently great sleep, I promise—you can too.

The End of the Book, but Not the End of Your Journey

"There is no real ending. It's just the place where you stop the story." — Frank Herbert

You've made it to the end. Not just to the end of the book, but to the beginning of something much better.

If you've come this far with me, first of all, thank you. Thank you for trusting me to walk alongside you through the tangled woods of sleepless nights, racing thoughts, nighttime anxiety, and everything else that steals our rest. Writing a book like this is a bit like tossing a message in a bottle into the ocean —you hope it finds the right people at the right time. If you're reading this, maybe you were one of them.

Now, let's be clear: the end of a book is not the end of your story. It's not even the end of your sleep journey. Real change happens not because you read about it, but because you decide to take a step. And then another. And another.

The truth is, building better sleep habits—and a better life—works a lot like hiking a long trail. You don't conquer it in a day. You don't always know what's around the next bend. Some days are beautiful. Some days are muddy. Some days you wonder why on earth you started this crazy trek at all.

But you keep going.

And somewhere along the way, you realize you've traveled farther than you ever thought you could.

That's my hope for you. That sleep, once your enemy, will become your ally. That rest will come easier. That the days will feel lighter, and the nights more peaceful. That you'll stop surviving and start thriving.

And when setbacks come—and they *will*—you'll know how to lace up your boots, shake off the dust, and keep moving forward.

In case no one has told you lately: you're doing better than you think you are. Change is already happening. The simple fact that you made it through this book means you are serious about reclaiming your life.

I couldn't be prouder of you.

Before I go, let me say one more thing. If we ever bump into each other on a hiking trail, at a coffee shop, or maybe even at a bookstore, I hope you'll stop and say hi. We've been on quite a journey together already, and it would be a pleasure to meet you in the real world too.

Until then, take what you've learned here. Make it yours. Make it work for you. And keep moving forward, even on the days when it feels slow and hard. Especially on those days.

I'll be cheering you on from my cozy quilted fortress of dreams.

Endless summer,
 Will

Bonus Chapter: What to Do When You STILL Can't Sleep

"Just because you turned the last page doesn't mean you're off the hook. Real change starts when the book closes."—Rogue Librarian Wisdom

First of all, if you're the type who flips straight to the end because you *just know* none of the stuff in the rest of the book will work for you—hi. Welcome. I see you.

But friend, you're like the person who eats dessert *before* dinner and then complains they're still hungry. Sure, this chapter is *delicious*, but if you skipped the main course (especially "Sleep Triage" —your real starting point), you're missing the meat and potatoes of fixing your sleep.

So if you haven't read the rest of the book, **stop right now**, flip yourself back to "Sleep Triage," and start there. Trust me—it's like trying to assemble Ikea furniture without the instructions if you don't. Only this time, the missing screw is your sanity.

Now, for the rest of you brave souls who *did* read the book and *still* find yourself staring at the ceiling like a philosophical goldfish, let's talk.

First, breathe. Seriously. Right now. If you're thinking, "Welp, I'm broken," let's pump the brakes on that train of thought. You're not broken. You're human. And sometimes, humans are stubborn creatures who don't change overnight just because a book told them to. (Shocking, I know.)

If you've had years—maybe decades—of rough sleep habits, it's going to take more than two weeks of good intentions and one sleepy-time tea to undo all that wiring. This is normal. This is okay. This is fixable.

Now comes the part where I lovingly push you out of the sleep nest and make you do the work.

Take a hard look at your setup. Is your sleep environment helping you or hurting you? You want cool, dark, quiet, and boring. Not blinking lights, not the hum of electronics, and definitely not the mystery smell from under the bed.

Have you eliminated the obvious villains? If caffeine, junky late-night snacks, a complete lack of exercise, or answering work emails at midnight are still hanging around like that one guest who doesn't know the party's over, it's time to kick them out.

Have you actually filled out your Sleep Routine Worksheet and stuck to it? (Not just read it and thought, *"Yeah, sounds good."*)

Are you giving your body enough movement during the day? If your biggest exercise was a vigorous scroll through social media, your body isn't ready to crash yet.

Did you let your brain wind down before bed? If your pre-bed ritual looks like three episodes of a true crime documentary followed by a TikTok binge, yeah. You're setting yourself up to be wide awake and wondering if your neighbors are serial killers.

You know what you need to do. Now, do it.

If you're still awake, good. That means you're still in the game.

Here's the secret sauce most people never tell you: the people who succeed at anything—sleep, weight loss, writing novels, tightrope walking—aren't the ones who never fail. They're the ones who keep experimenting.

Getting great sleep is just like anything else worth doing. You try things. You notice what works and what doesn't. You tweak. You learn. You keep going.

That's it. That's the whole "secret."

Think about people who lose weight and keep it off. They didn't just follow one magic diet—they tried things. They cut out foods that didn't work for them. They stole good ideas from different plans. They figured out what made *their* body tick.

Your sleep is the same way.

You are not doomed. You are not exempt. You are not too far gone. You are a person in process. And you, my friend, are closer than you think.

Here's your new mission, should you choose to accept it (and you should): keep experimenting with what works. Ruthlessly eliminate what doesn't. Build the best sleep environment you can. Stick with the basics from this book. Give yourself time. Keep going.

If you're awake at 2 AM, don't spiral. Don't tell yourself, *"I'll never fix this."* Instead, go back to your toolkit. Get up if you're not sleepy after 20 minutes. Use the Military Method. Stretch, breathe, pray, journal—whatever works to reset your mind. Trust the process. And tomorrow, recommit.

Sleep is something you allow, not something you wrestle to the ground.

This whole book wasn't about handing you a magic wand. It was about handing you the tools and saying, "Here. Build something better."

And you can.

You already are.

Stay patient. Stay curious. Stay determined. Sleep will come. You're not chasing some mythical beast —you're just rebuilding something your body already knows how to do.

I'm cheering you on. You've got this. Now go get some sleep.

(And if you ever need a reminder... Hey, I wrote this whole book just for you.)

Works Cited

Ackerman, D. (n.d.). *Sleep With Me* [Podcast]. Sleep With Me Podcast. https://www.sleepwithmepodcast.com/

American College of Physicians. (2016). Cognitive behavioral therapy for insomnia: Recommendation statement. *Annals of Internal Medicine, 165*(2), 125–133. https://doi.org/10.7326/M15-2175

Centers for Disease Control and Prevention. (2022). Sleep and sleep disorders. https://www.cdc.gov/sleep/index.html

Ferracioli-Oda E, Qawasmi A, Bloch MH. Meta-analysis: melatonin for the treatment of primary sleep disorders. PLoS One. 2013 May 17;8(5):e63773. doi: 10.1371/journal.pone.0063773. PMID: 23691095; PMCID: PMC3656905. https://pmc.ncbi.nlm.nih.gov/articles/PMC3656905/

Field, T. (2010). Touch for socioemotional and physical well-being: A review. *Developmental Review, 30*(4), 367–383.

Kalmbach, D. A., Arnedt, J. T., Pillai, V., & Ciesla, J. A. (2015). The impact of sleep on female sexual response and desire. *Journal of Sexual Medicine, 12*(5), 1221–1231.

Lastella, M., O'Mullan, C., Paterson, J. L., & Reynolds, A. C. (2019). Sex and sleep: Perceptions of sex as a sleep-promoting behavior in the general adult population. *Frontiers in Public Health, 7*, 33.

Leproult, R., & Van Cauter, E. (2011). Effect of one week of sleep restriction on testosterone levels in young healthy men. *JAMA, 305*(21), 2173–2174.

National Institutes of Health. (2023). Cognitive behavioral therapy for insomnia (CBT-I). National Center for Complementary and Integrative Health. https://www.nccih.nih.gov/health/insomnia

The Guardian. (2024, November 4). Is it true that the blue light from night-time scrolling can stop you sleeping? *The Guardian.* https://www.theguardian.com/lifeandstyle/2024/nov/04/is-it-true-that-the-blue-light-from-night-time-scrolling-can-stop-you-sleeping

U.S. Food and Drug Administration. (2014–2022). Drug approvals and database for suvorexant (Belsomra), lemborexant (Dayvigo), daridorexant (Quviviq). https://www.fda.gov/drugs

About the author

After 35 years as a teacher, librarian, administrator, coach, and professional wearer of many hats (some more stylish than others), I did what every weary educator dreams of during standardized testing week: I retired.

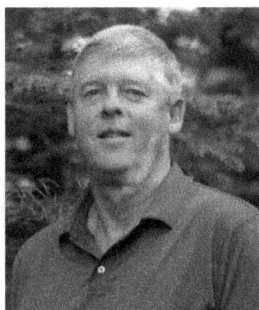

But let's be clear—retirement for me wasn't a surrender to rocking chairs and reruns. It was more of a personal commencement ceremony. While my students tossed caps in the air, I tossed my briefcase in the closet and asked myself, "Whatta ya wanna do today?"

My answer: everything.

Armed with six decades of stories, scars, and a slightly overstuffed backpack, I headed to the woods —not in the sit-and-muse-like-Thoreau sense, but the hike-from-Lake-Huron-to-Lake-Michigan kind of way. I wanted to live deliberately, seek the essential, and wring every drop of meaning from this next chapter.

Before all that, I served students across Michigan and China as an English and Spanish teacher, librarian, basketball coach, alternative ed principal, tech trainer, preschool director, and district administrator.

I've taught in classrooms, coached on courts, and even co-wrangled an 800-kid preschool program (no small feat, trust me).

My formal credentials include a B.A. in English/Spanish, a Master's in Library and Information Science, and a certificate in Educational Technology—but most of my real education has come from the trail, the classroom, and the occasional parenting misadventure.

Today, I'm a writer, traveler, speaker, and perpetual learner. I write books, build online resources, hike long trails, and help people wrestle meaning out of life's chaos.

Whether I'm creating tools to help hikers prepare for the backcountry, guides to help readers sleep better, or humorous tales from my years in education, my goal is the same: leave the world a little more inspired—and maybe a little better rested—than I found it. I believe the best chapters are still ahead. Let's walk there together.

Also by Will Swartz

▌ **The Rogue Librarian's Guide to Falling Asleep in 2 Minutes—Starting Tonight (Rogue Rapid Reads)**
The streamlined, no-fluff version of the full sleep book. Perfect for those who want quick wins and straight-up sleep solutions without reading a dissertation. It's like the CliffsNotes of better sleep—with jokes.

▌ **A Walk Across Michigan: Hiking the Shore-to-Shore Trail from Lake Huron to Lake Michigan**
Part trail journal, part history lesson, part love letter to the woods—and all heart. Join me on a hike across the mitten state, with a backpack full of stories, unexpected wisdom, and maybe a few blisters. Michigan's natural beauty and forgotten past get a spotlight here.

▌ **The Trail Quiz: 47 Vital Questions You Need to Answer Before Going on a Longer Trail**
Thinking about hiking a longer trail? Start here. This guide is like having a sarcastic but helpful trail buddy who asks all the right questions (so you don't end up cold, wet, or halfway up a mountain without coffee). Includes practical advice, real talk, and trail-tested wisdom.

▌ **Kids Elf Tracker: 25 Days of Elf Antics, Ratings, and Holiday Fun**
Part logbook, part activity book, all joy. This delightful holiday companion helps kids (and parents) track the daily adventures of their Elf on the Shelf. Includes silly scoring, creative prompts, and enough giggles to get you through December with your sanity mostly intact.

📘 How I Trained ChatGPT to Write Like Me — And How You Can Too!

For writers, creators, and curious tech explorers — this guide pulls back the curtain on training AI to match your voice (without sounding like a robot lawyer from 1998). If you've ever wondered how to co-write with ChatGPT and make it sound like you — not like "Generic Internet Person #453" — this book's for you.

These are available in a variety of formats (Print, ebook & audio) at:

https://linktr.ee/wswartz